Researching
Trust and Health

Routledge Studies in Health and Social Welfare

1. Researching Trust and Health
Edited by Julie Brownlie, Alexandra
Greene and Alexandra Howson

Researching
Trust and Health

Edited by
Julie Brownlie,
Alexandra Greene
and
Alexandra Howson

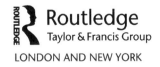
Routledge
Taylor & Francis Group

LONDON AND NEW YORK

First published 2008 by Routledge
2 Park Square, Milton Park, Abingdon, Oxon OX14 4RN
52 Vanderbilt Avenue, New York, NY 10017

Routledge is an imprint of the Taylor & Francis Group, an informa business

First issued in paperback 2012

© 2008 Taylor & Francis

All rights reserved. No part of this book may be reprinted or reproduced or utilised in any form or by any electronic, mechanical, or other means, now known or hereafter invented, including photocopying and recording, or in any information storage or retrieval system, without permission in writing from the publishers.

Trademark Notice: Product or corporate names may be trademarks or registered trade-marks, and are used only for identification and explanation without intent to infringe.

Library of Congress Cataloging-in-Publication Data

Researching trust and health / edited by Julie Brownlie, Alexandra Greene, and Alexandra Howson.
    p. ; cm. — (Routledge studies in health and social welfare ; 1)
    Includes bibliographical references and index.
    ISBN-13: 978-0-415-95851-6 (hardback : alk. paper)
    ISBN-10: 0-415-95851-2 (hardback : alk. paper) 1. Medical ethics. 2. Medical personnel and patient. 3. Trust. I. Brownlie, Julie. II. Greene, Alexandra. III. Howson, Alexandra. IV. Series.
    [DNLM: 1. Nurse-Patient Relations. 2. Interprofessional Relations. 3. Nursing Care. 4. Research Design. 5. Trust. WY 87 R432 2008]
    R725.5.R47 2008
    174.2—dc22   2007042983

ISBN13: 978-0-415-64310-1 (pbk)
ISBN13: 978-0-415-95851-6 (hbk)
ISBN13: 978-0-203-92827-1 (ebk)

Contents

Foreword

At the time of writing this foreword, having read a draft of this fine volume, I am following the media coverage of the trial of a nurse in Germany who has killed several patients in the famous Berlin hospital Charité. Through her crimes she has not only betrayed most horribly the trust of her victims but also the trust that their relatives, her colleagues and her employer vested in her. Because she is a representative of her organization, her profession and the health care system, her case stirs the public mood and raises specific questions about the circumstances of these murders as well as more general questions about trust in health care contexts. How could she do it?

Answers to this question have to address different levels of analysis: the nurse's personality, competence, motivation and attitude towards life and death; her social networks of relationships with family, friends, patients, visitors, colleagues, superiors; the organizational and institutional systems in which she was working; and her general place in society. When we try to understand what it means to trust and be trusted, all these levels matter, and a particular strength of this volume is that it takes the multilayered nature of trust very seriously.

When we imagine ourselves in the position of the above-mentioned nurse's patients, the issue of vulnerability is particularly salient. The concept of health entails the possibility of the loss of good health and the vulnerability of human life, both of which are primordial experiences of human existence. The term vulnerability originates from the Latin word *vulnus*, which means wound. More abstract uses of the term nowadays still carry this original meaning of externally caused injury.

Yet it is because health and vulnerability are so strongly connected and also emotionally charged that we have to be extra careful when discussing trust in the context of health. We have to distinguish clearly between the general threat of suffering from an injury or illness for which no-one else is to blame and the harm that can be done by those to whom we entrust the injured and the sick. The murderous nurse was not responsible for her patients' severe conditions in the first place, but she outrageously ended their lives instead of helping to save them. This is not a trivial point. When people go to see a dentist, do they fear the pain the treatment normally involves or the pain the dentist might unnecessarily cause them? Only the latter is a question of trust. In other words, trust in health care is not primarily about being cured but about the competent and benevolent efforts that are made to cure. Trust in health care is broken when such efforts are expected and possible but not forthcoming due to individual, organizational or institutional weaknesses and failures. In this book, the contributors recognize that trust concerns specifically the vulnerability that results from people's dependence on the social world around them. This basic insight gains a certain sense of urgency when health is at stake.

A further clarification concerns an important precondition whereby it only makes sense to speak of trust when it is possible to identify a 'trustor' and a 'trustee' to whom we can attribute agency, that is, some autonomy and accountability in their placing and honouring of trust (or not). Again, this may seem a trivial point, but it promotes the precision and relevance of analyzing trust in the context of health care. For example, unless they are unconscious or totally ignorant, patients themselves decide whether they trust or distrust a doctor, a hospital, a health insurance company and so on, even when they have no choice which doctor, hospital or insurance to use. In their trust, they are influenced by their environment in many ways, but the trust or distrust is still theirs. In return, the trustees, for example doctors, exercise agency in honouring their patients' trust, but in so doing they also have to operate within limitations that they did not choose themselves and that are therefore not attributable to their own trustworthiness.

In any discussion of trust, we need to specify the trustors and trustees and how much agency they are assumed to have. This is not always easy in the context of health care, which is characterized by a high degree of "systemness" where agency is highly distributed and depersonalized. Did the nurse or the system kill the patients in Berlin? And who trusted the nurse (or the system) too much? The studies in this book do a very good job in connecting the discussion of trust to fairly concrete trustors and trustees who do have agency. And in some cases authors prefer to speak of confidence instead of trust when they refer to expectations towards an abstract system that is not really a trustee in itself.

If trust is about recognizing and accepting human agency, then it is not surprising that breaches of trust often trigger attempts to curb this agency through tighter control. The bureaucratic control-reflex that typically follows dramatic cases and scandals, such as the recent Charité killings in Germany and various well-publicized scandals in the United Kingdom, is evidence for the societal suspicion of agency and the institutionalization of distrust in modern societies. One of the remarkable features of this book is that it moves beyond the old trust–control dichotomy and frames trust and control as a duality. This means that policies introducing greater accountability and more standardized performance-measures in health care can be understood in their ambivalent effect of potentially promoting and destroying trust. It also implies the realization that control depends on trust, so that the introduction of new control measures requires trust in those who design and apply the measures. Therefore, at best, this merely shifts the trust problem to another level—down to users or up to regulators. Human agency, as an opportunity and a threat, cannot be eliminated. This is reflected in the studies in this volume. They recognize that trust-building is about finding ways of positively accepting agency and limiting it without destroying it, even if this leaves room for murderous nurses.

Finally, the agency of trustors and trustees points to the irreducible uncertainty that surrounds our vulnerability. In my own research on trust, I have concluded that trust requires a leap of faith by which this uncertainty is suspended, and positive expectations towards the actions and intentions of others become possible. The notion of the leap of faith is superficially accepted in many areas of trust research but at the same time fairly hard to pin down in empirical cases. It is interesting that in the context of health care, vulnerability and uncertainty seem to be so pronounced that leaps of faith are much more evident here.

It remains a methodological challenge to identify concrete instances of such suspension, but in many interviews reported in this volume we find accounts of people who look for good reasons and who try to anchor their decisions but who also, at some point, just do it, stop worrying and manage to live as if everything will be fine. Inasmuch as the accounts are about the ways in which people deal with the agency of others in relation to whom they are vulnerable, they offer important insights to trust research. In the context of health care, it appears to be second nature for us to accept that leaps of faith do not eliminate vulnerability and uncertainty but make them tolerable. Some nurses may always be able to kill patients and get away with it, yet trust emphasizes the fact that almost all nurses will not abuse their agency but use it positively to offer help and support.

The leaps of faith that enable trust are ultimately to be understood as emotional commitments and accomplishments. I trace this back, for example, to the classic works of William James on the will to believe, and to more recent writings by Jack Barbalet, who developed a similar understanding in parallel to my own efforts. It implies that trust is idiosyncratic and resides fundamentally with individuals who cannot be forced to reach the state of trust. All the more, it is important to analyze—as many studies in this volume do—how individuals are not isolated in their trust but deeply embedded in social networks, organizational structures and institutional frameworks.

This edited volume deals with a topic that social scientists have come across before, even when they have no specific interest in health care, because many core contributions on the nature of modern societies have used the trust problem in health care to focus or illustrate their points. As examples, I mention Talcott Parsons, Niklas Luhmann and Anthony Giddens, all of whom have been concerned with the relationship between lay persons and professional experts; the systems behind these relationships; and the social interaction connecting the interpersonal level and the system-level. In the same way that these authors have used the topic of health care to illustrate more general theoretical arguments, this book offers theoretical insights beyond our immediate concerns about trust in concrete contemporary health care contexts and beyond topical scandals too.

In my own book on trust, I encouraged trust researchers in other disciplines such as management and economics to pay more attention to the research on trust in the sociology of health and medicine. With the publication of this excellent collection of conceptual and empirical contributions, it will now be hard for any trust researcher to ignore this field of inquiry. It is particularly refreshing that the research reported here breaks out of the moulds that have been shaping trust research in other areas. In particular, I am sure that many readers will appreciate the qualitative methods used and the sensitivity to process, richness and reflexivity in this book as much as I do. Of course, those who study trust in health care contexts should also build on the extensive research on trust conducted in other areas; but the exploratory tone of many of the findings presented here is not at all a signal, to me, that research on trust in health care is still at the beginning and trying to catch up. Rather, it is an indication of the cutting-edge quality of the researchers' use of sophisticated concepts and methods instead of crude, simplistic tools that mutilate the phenomenon of trust.

As a final reminder that this book deals with a classic problem of human societies and not some faddish issues that will be gone tomorrow, I would like to mention the Hippocratic Oath that was established in ancient Greece in the fourth century BC. We can interpret it as a way of dealing with the problem of trust in health care in that it recognizes the vulnerability of patients and aims to establish a professional institutional standard while not denying the substantial agency of all the actors involved in health care. Nowadays, we still seem to be dealing with the same problems, but the editors of this volume have to be congratulated on presenting us with an up-to-date set of questions—and with answers—in the light of the truly serious and specific issues we face in our health care systems today.

Guido Möllering
(Cologne, 2 July 2007)

Acknowledgments

We would like to thank Ben Holtzman for his editorial guidance, our anonymous reviewers for their helpful comments and Irene Anderson for her careful reading and generous advice. Similarly, our thanks to Jennifer Waterton for her excellent indexing work, to Claire Murray for her wonderful job of formatting, and to the University of Aberdeen for financial and administrative support.

Introduction

BACKGROUND

There is a great deal of talk about trust: what it is, how to nurture it, and if it is lost, how to retrieve it. Its similarity to love has been noted in recent writings: both concepts are used promiscuously and, as a result are difficult to pin down (Solomon 2000). Indeed, in literature at least, trust comes second only to love as a plotline (Hardin 2002, 31). But the lively global debate, both inside and outside academia about the nature of trust and the conditions necessary to establish and sustain it, suggests that in 'real life,' trust may now even have usurped, or at least caught up with, love as our primary focus. The message from politicians, the media, academics, pollsters, practitioners and that most mythical of entities, 'the public,' is that trust matters. It is somewhat surprising, then, to find that the concept of trust is still widely used in an unquestioning or unproblematic way. Even though politicians and pollsters might get away with treating trust as a 'primitive term'—something that we know when we see it—(Hardin 2001, 8), the job of social scientists has been to investigate what comprises trust and how and where it is practised. Although teasing out trust's nature—for example, its cognitive and affective dimensions (Lewis and Weigert 1985)—is beginning to happen, there are still few published accounts exploring trust empirically (Möllering 2005; Bijlsma-Frankema and Klein Woolthius 2005) and, even fewer in relation to health (for exceptions see Lee-Treweek 2002; Brownlie and Howson 2005, 2006; Entwistle and Quick 2006).

The editors of this volume—two sociologists and an anthropologist—began thinking about trust some years ago in the context of health-related research (e.g., cervical screening participation, child immunization, diabetes management). The idea for an edited collection came from our realization that, though we knew many people working on trust issues in relation to health, and although there was a literature that discussed trust in abstract terms, there was little available material we could draw on for our own work that specifically addressed trust in relation to health. As Rowe and Calnan (2006a, 392) observed recently in relation to the United Kingdom, empirical research on trust and relationships in health care is 'urgently needed.' At the same time, as researchers, we were also increasingly aware of the paucity of methodological discussion in relation to trust. Yet, as the contributions to this volume make clear, the issue of trust is at the heart of people's experiences in relation to health care organization and delivery, and there is, therefore, a need to begin to share our stories about researching trust in this context.

In the remainder of this introduction, by way of background, we delineate further this relationship between health and trust; we offer an overview of the chapters; and we highlight some emergent issues around researching trust in general and in relation to the particular studies in this volume. We conclude by reviewing what it means to research technologies and rationalities of health and trust. There are always gaps in such collections, and this one is no exception, so before making a proper start, it might be useful if we offered a word or two about what the book is *not*. It is not the final word on research methodologies relating to trust, not least because, as we explain in more detail later, our focus is very much on qualitative research. Similarly, although trust has emerged as a key concept across a range of (inter)disciplinary areas, including most notably organizational studies (Connell and Mannion 2006) and psychology (Das and Teng 2004), the emphasis in this book is shaped by perspectives in sociology, medical anthropology and health studies. There are other absences: most significantly, though we have drawn on contributors from North America, the United Kingdom and Scandinavia, work on trust and health within developing countries is not addressed. This is an increasingly significant area of research (Gilson 2006), with trust in low-income countries now identified as having a potentially key role in reducing the marginalization and vulnerability of the poor (Connell and Mannion 2006). The present collection, along with other texts looking at research in high-income nations, usefully serves as a point of comparison.

RELATING TRUST AND HEALTH

Health crucially affords specific analytical opportunities in relation to trust, not least because at an interpersonal, institutional and system level, health practices depend on trust relations. Why should this be so? Most researchers who are interested in health and trust are agreed that the answer to this question reflects a complicated bundle of realities. At a micro or interpersonal level, these include: the uncertainties that mark health issues; the risks attached to professional competencies; the asymmetry of the relationship between health professionals and patients; and the associated vulnerability of the patient as a result of the interplay between some or all of these factors (Connell and Mannion 2006; Calnan and Rowe 2006). Vulnerability has become central to how trust generally is understood and is particularly to the fore when we feel unwell or when we are told we are sick. Researching trust and health in tandem, then, telescopes this relationship between trust and vulnerability but also, crucially, as we discuss later, the connections between trust, vulnerability and emotions.

Trust, like health, becomes more visible, then, once its taken-for-grantedness is ruptured. Naming the inextricable 'helplessness' (Möllering 2006, 3) attached to trust might be akin to naming the elephant in the room, but the irony is that it is through leaving this vulnerability unnamed or unsaid that trust happens in the first place. At an interpersonal level in relation to health, trust facilitates the successful delivery of health care, and trusting patient–provider relations have the potential to deliver direct therapeutic benefit (Mechanic 1998; see Cook and Stepanikova, this volume). Indeed, because of its forward-looking nature, trust may be a more sensitive indicator of performance in these relationships than patient satisfaction (Thom, Hall and Pawlson 2004).

At a macrolevel, trust matters in relation to health because health care is a deeply sociopolitical issue (even in countries where health care is largely privatized, as in the United States). A decline of trust in health organizations, the argument goes, undermines trust in the state more generally, and this, in turn, impacts on economic security and the ability of administrations to govern democratically (Robb and Greenhalgh 2006). In other words, trust in health care contributes to wider societal values and norms that form the basis for further ethical outcomes such as fair distribution of resources (Gilson 2006). Although some might suggest we are asking too much of trust for it to maintain social order in this way and point instead to other features that aid cooperation, including incentives (Cook, Hardin and Levi 2005), others continue to see trust as a form of social glue—the means, following Luhmann (1979), of dealing with social complexity and avoiding the paralysis such complexity might induce. Recent North American texts—*The Trust Prescription for Health Care* and *The Trust Crisis in Health Care* (Shore 2005, 2007)—have signalled the centrality of trust for health care economics, captured in Shore's maxim that 'the organization that owns trust owns its marketplace' (2007, 8). But the wider argument is that because of their fundamental relevance to the social fabric, 'trust matters' are not just an issue for the health marketplace of neoliberal economies but are of worldwide concern. The potential here, then, is that the sustenance or restoration of trust in health care could temper some of the negative consequences of recent social changes more generally (Gilson 2006; Illingworth 2005).

It is debates such as these about why trust matters at a micro and macro-level in relation to health that have provoked the question: should health be considered a specific case for thinking about trust? (Gilson 2006). In this collection, we look to health as a means of illuminating trust and, at the same time, we draw on trust to understand health. We position health as a key, yet under-researched, area which is deserving of analytical attention in its own right in relation to trust *and* as a way of exploring some of the wider social changes that have foregrounded trust generally in policy, practice and theory in recent years.

This collection tackles the issue of trust at an interpersonal level: in relationships between lay people and professionals; between health professionals themselves; and between providers and managers in health care contexts. Even though the focus on trust between professionals has been identified as a significant under-researched area in relation to trust and health for some time, much research remains focused on the experiences of lay participants rather than on practitioner or managerial/organisational perspectives (Brownlie and Howson 2005; Calnan and Rowe 2006). Hall (2006) has argued that, in a U.S. context, one reason for this focus is the emphasis on being able to choose relationships with one's own physician and the market-based nature of health care provision. Yet, as Rowe and Calnan (2006b) make clear, trust relationships will vary depending on models of health care delivery and cultural assumptions about health in different countries. Personal trust, then, might have greater significance in market-based systems like that of the United States, whereas in tax-financed systems such as the United Kingdom and Norway, public trust might have a more prominent role. Shore (2005) notes that, in fact, the United States does not have a health care 'system' as such—it has a collection of provider organizations and payers that are fragmented and often in competition with each other. What he describes as a set of 'multiple dichotomies'—physicians versus hospitals, providers versus payers, government versus providers—constitutes, then, a very specific setting for thinking about trust. Cook and Stepanikova in this volume note that it may be too early to say if their finding of a relative paucity of evidence on health care outcomes of generalized forms of trust in health care providers 'is an artefact of a research niche that is still immature or whether it reflects a true lack of significant relationships between these forms of trust and health care outcomes.'

The key point we are making here, however, is that whatever the cultural context, health and trust have become key sites for thinking through the changing role of professions and the notion of professionalism (Kuhlmann 2006). The assumption that relationships between practitioners, or between practitioners and managers, in health contexts are not problematic, or at least do not impact on care, is increasingly questioned (Calnan, Rowe and Entwistle 2006, 479). One of the premises of this collection is that the interconnectivity of lay people, practitioners, managers and policymakers makes it artificial to consider any of these relationships in isolation. As the studies in this volume make clear across different contexts, even when we think we are trusting just one person, we, and the person in whom we invest our trust, are embedded in a network of interpersonal, institutional and system relations. This is particularly true where health care systems involve many organizations and multiple sets of individuals working within them (Gilson 2006). As Luhmann notes (1979, 53), drawing on the case of thalidomide, this network of relations carries particular implications when thinking about trust because 'It is often the case that someone transmits authentically, but he is only the last link in a long chain of information processing'.

A key thematic concern of this volume is this multilayered nature of trust, which we began to conceptualize in our earlier work on immunization (Brownlie and Howson 2005, 2006). Relationships between interpersonal, institutional and system levels in health contexts are often underspecified, as is how these relationships are shaped by social changes. It also needs to be noted that intrapersonal trust, although not the focus of this collection, is, whether we choose to theorize it in a more or less social way, unavoidably a component of all these layers, as it is the site at which they are inevitably worked through, consciously or otherwise. Some have argued that a sociologically informed perspective allows for this layered approach to be used to investigate trust both within specific settings and in relation to wider sociopolitical contexts (Simmel 1950, 1990; Möllering 2006; Brownlie and Howson 2005), and concomitantly, to explore trust within particular relationships, such as those between health practitioners, or health practitioners and patients, or between public health organisations and the community in general. Thus, one of the aims of this collection is to consolidate these different levels of analysis to inform the broader theoretical objective of thinking about trust as a multilayered concept and, concurrently, to draw on empirically based research, to unravel its complexity and hence support stakeholders in the health arena. In order to do this, and to address questions of how, why and where trust has gained prominence across health practices, theoretical claims about the nature of trust—both generally and specifically in relation to health—need to be interrogated. We turn to this task in the next chapter but before doing so, in the remainder of this introduction, we briefly explain the structure of the book, outline the contents of the chapters to follow and offer some comment on the challenges of researching trust.

BOOK STRUCTURE AND CHAPTER OVERVIEW

There are ten chapters in this volume. The first chapter explores the conceptual context of the volume as a whole. In it, we review those aspects of recent analyses of the nature of trust that we believe are key to understanding the relationship between health and trust. In particular, we investigate the shifting relationships between interpersonal, institutional and public trust; the sociopolitical context of trust; and a conceptual frame for understanding these changes based on the relationship between trust and confidence. Three further issues—power, distrust and the social differentiation of trust—which are woven through the nine remaining chapters are then highlighted. We have grouped these chapters into three sections. The first explores the multidimensional nature of trust primarily from the perspective of users and the second, mainly, from the viewpoint of practitioners. The final section looks at the role of community (ies) in debates about trust and health and also engages with the notion of social capital and its relationship to trust and health outcomes. The division of interpersonal, institutional and social trust might have been a more obvious structure but would have undermined what is, in effect, one of the key messages of the collection: the nonsensicality of thinking about these layers except in relation to each other. Nevertheless, the division remains somewhat heuristic not least, of course, because the levels of analysis we have chosen to structure the volume around are necessarily also interwoven. Concomitantly, the contributors have, in the main, chosen to peg their substantive concerns on 'lay,' 'practitioner' or 'community' issues, and so we have taken this as our starting point for exploring the multilayered nature of trust.

The first chapter grouping, then, engages with this from the perspective of what can broadly be seen as users of health services. In Parr and Davidson's study, these are users of electronic support groups (ESGs); in Solbjør's research, they are women who have participated in breast screening programs in Norway; and in Sheach Leith's case, the users are parents in the United Kingdom whose children's organs and tissues were retained after post-mortems. Drawing on published first-hand accounts of virtual health communities, Parr and Davidson foreground the voices of individuals with anxiety disorders and more general mental health problems. These individuals share 'real-world' experiences of extreme social and spatial exclusion as a result of debilitating emotional and affective disorders. By exploring circulations of trust in the virtual world through ESGs, the authors address questions of location, using sociogeographical insights to interrogate the potential significance of *where* trustful relations might take place. Participants in Parr and Davidson's research describe profound difficulties with physically situated support groups that require their bodily presence in spaces that are communicatively demanding and immediately emotionally charged. The chapter examines the nature of emotional involvement and detachment that is possible online, and by thinking through the distances and proximities that constitute trust in virtual worlds, as they are specifically configured through questions of emotional and mental health, the authors illuminate new ways of thinking through the problems and possibilities of trustful and caring relations. In particular, they argue for further exploration of the performativity of virtual trust relations, given that in contemporary health care contexts, 'many of us trust non-proximate, unseen peers, more readily than "real-life" practitioners.'

Solbjør's chapter focuses on mammography as a visualizing technology that makes it especially interesting to explore whether and how technological aspects and expertise influence participation in, and trust of, the screening program. Her chapter offers an empirical analysis of focus group interviews that explores mammography technology, expertise and visualization as connected to women's trust in mammography screening. As her analysis makes plain, trusting may occur because the technology associated with mammography offers a sense of objectivity. But mammography does not work by itself, it requires experts to handle it and interpret the results. The experiences of the women in Solbjør's study suggest that trust in expert knowledge coexists with knowledge of the potential for error (in particular false negatives), and this act of trusting may be associated with the way that visualization is privileged within the diagnostic rubric of mammography screening.

Drawing on documentary data produced in the wake of the organ retention scandal in the United Kingdom, Sheach Leith explores the steps taken ostensibly to restore trust in relation to a distinct facet of health care during a period of acute flux. Her chapter explores the complexity of the trust relationships highlighted by the organ retention scandal and surveys the extent to which the perceived crisis in trust can be restored through the implementation of informed consent. In doing so, she lays the groundwork for analyzing the significance of other discourses, namely the gift relationship and *post-mortem citizenship* and argues that consideration of the wider sociopolitical context in which consent is obtained is crucial to a full understanding of the trust relationships embedded within post-mortem practice, and the potential restoration of trust.

The second section, also allows for users' voices but draws predominantly on the perspectives of health practitioners. In Greene, McKiernan and Greene's study, these include a range of health professionals based at diabetes outpatient clinics; in Huby's chapter, health professionals involved in integrated health and social care settings; and in Guthrie's research, GPs working in primary care settings. Greene et al.'s focus on trust is informed by diabetes in secondary care; rising mortality and morbidity associated with poor management of diabetes; and a greater emphasis on high-quality services for children and young people. The chapter examines young people's and health professionals' experiences of working together in seven outpatient clinics in Scotland and describes how a powerful ideology portraying teenagers as deviant and risk-taking, and therefore untrustworthy, appears to clash with the ethos in the National Health Service of improving trust between health professionals and patients. An advantage of this analysis is that it also draws on a study undertaken 10 years earlier with many of the same health professionals (albeit with a different cohort of young people). The interviews reveal changes in the stories that health professionals are telling today, and their approach explores how better understandings of trust between young people and health professionals might be developed to support young people's optimal self-management of diabetes and corresponding long-term health. Drawing on anthropological work on the nature of reciprocity, the authors interpret the good relations between various clinics and between patients and health professionals as key gifting relationships. These relationships, they argue, are based on networking and the exchange of information, support, gossip and anxieties (Mauss 1993) and are key to delivering altruistic care: a form of care where everyone's contribution is valued and where trust is built on the basis of good faith rather than sanctions. This study, informed by the health practitioners' and young people's voices, suggests there is a misfit between such notions of care, trust and reciprocity and the new audit culture.

Huby's chapter, building this time on Garfinkel's (1967) ethnomethodological insight that how people account for themselves—and the way these accounts are then interpreted and understood—is at the heart of our 'taken-for-granted' trust in the social order, develops the focus on accountability which was highlighted by Greene et al. She does this by examining how systems of accountability rebound in various ways on the social construction of trust in the context of 'integrated' health care in Scotland. Although there is a growing interest in accountability and the construction and erosion of trust between providers and users of health care, less is known about how trust is constructed, maintained or undermined in relationships among staff, and how systems of accountability impact on these relationships. Huby's chapter focuses on the latter, and through exploring the concept of 'care pathways' in two different health settings, draws general implications for the ways in which the relationship between accountability and trust among practitioners may be managed in health care settings undergoing reorganization.

Turning to trust in the relationship between general practitioners (GPs) and patients, Guthrie's chapter unfolds against the background of regulatory reforms in the United Kingdom, which were introduced to reduce the risk of system or individual failure, but which are widely perceived as having been corrosive of public and patient faith in medicine. This reflects Huby's and Greene et al.'s analyses of the ways in which 'audit society' mechanisms (Power 1997) act to undermine trust (O'Neill 2002). One response from organized medicine has been to reaffirm the importance of 'professionalism' by promoting new models of the social contract between doctors and society. Such a contract places emphasis on doctors learning to trust patients to play a major part in technical decisions. Yet, as Guthrie observes, this change in the direction of trusting will be a painful process for many doctors, as it requires them to cede at least some professional expertise. To unpack aspects of this key relationship between trust and expertise, Guthrie draws on the asymmetrical claims to legitimacy made by doctors and patients.

The final section of the volume shifts the focus not only onto the role of community (ies) in debates about trust and health but also engages with the notion of social capital and its relationship to trust and health outcomes. In Haddow and Cunningham-Burley's chapter, the community in question is made up of different social groupings, each with particular views on the development of a large-scale genetic databank in Scotland. Law's study, based on an analysis of one community's opposition to the citing of a cellular phone tower (or mast as it is known in the U.K.), offers a critique of the relationship between health, trust and social capital. Cook and Stepanikova's chapter, meanwhile, returns to this relationship between social capital, health and trust but engages with the issue of the health outcomes of trust in the U.S. context, highlighting again the differentiated nature of trust.

In their chapter on large-scale genetic databases, Haddow and Cunningham-Burley examine the issue of public trust and the mistrust in expert and abstract systems that arises from the risks associated with technological developments. Their study focuses on Generation Scotland, an organization that aims to create an ethically sound, population-based infrastructure to identify the genetic basis of common complex diseases such as cancer, stroke, heart disease and mental health problems. Generation Scotland incorporates several partners and seeks to engender trust by involving the public through consultation. Haddow and Cunningham-Burley consider the extent to which public consultation about genetic databases can both influence the institutional constraints of science and encourage reflective practice amongst all those involved in the development and use of genetic databases for health research. As the authors argue, uncertainty about risks generates mistrust and leads to demands for heightened regulation and surveillance but also furthers dependence on abstract systems. This pairing of uncertainty and mistrust, or the 'problem of trust,' is increasingly acknowledged in science/society relations—for instance, policy documents, and other arenas where the institutions of science confront their publics, reproduce a mantra of a lack of trust or confidence in, techno-science. Consequently, public understanding of, and engagement in, science is invoked as a corrective to a perceived corrosion of trust. Though the need to build public confidence and trust, often through 'consultation,' is seen as paramount, Haddow and Cunningham-Burley caution against a view of a homogeneous public as either having or withholding trust. Instead they emphasize—through an analysis of a public consultation focused on whether and where there is mistrust, and in what contexts and for what reasons—a more contextual, experiential and ambivalent picture of trust.

Taking issue with the claim that enhanced wellbeing and health are among the most welcome side effects of social capital, Alex Law draws from a case study of a local grassroots campaign against a cellular phone tower to show how the idea of 'cultures of challenge' in health movements dispute Robert Putnam's (2004) notion of social trust as essentially consensual and prepolitical. His case study did not begin with an explicit focus on questions of trust and mistrust, but they soon emerged as crucial variables. Stakeholders were highly conscious of being seen as 'trustworthy' even while they played a tactical game to outmaneuver their opponents. Returning again to this theme of the relationship between knowledge/expertise and trust—raised, too, by Solbjør and by Parr and Davidson—Law argues his findings reflect the shifting scales of trust characteristic of modernity:

from those inscribed in face-to-face community relationships to abstract and unseen sociotechnical systems, populated by anonymous experts. In his chapter on health movements that present cultures of challenge, Law problematizes Giddens' idea of 'active trust' in experts through exploring, at a community level, scepticism in establishment expertise. Yet, as he goes on to argue, this is necessarily a qualified critique as often this scepticism is itself based on other claims to expert knowledge.

Building on the argument that relationships between different kinds of trust are not well understood, Karen Cook and Irena Stepanikova explore how health care access, quality and related health care outcomes are linked to interpersonal and generalized trust. The types of trust they focus on include trust between patients and physicians, trust or confidence in the medical system and institutions, and trust inherent in patients' networks outside of health care environments. Arguing that the decision to seek health care is partially determined by the level of an individual's trust in providers and, more broadly, in medical institutions, they summarize evidence consistent with the argument that a link exists between trust and health care outcomes. These authors review the existing empirical evidence to provide a more comprehensive picture of how various forms of trust relate to health care outcomes and to propose an empirical model of health care outcomes of trust. This model can serve as a base for further empirical research and theoretical development on the topic of trust and health care, as well as a useful tool in the applied realm of policies and interventions intended to improve health care outcomes.

TRUSTING RESEARCH

From the discussion so far it is clear that, at a conceptual level, rich debates are beginning to emerge about trust in relation to health. Although, since the 1990s, a body of empirical research on trust has begun to develop (see Möllering 2006 for an overview of trust methodologies), within health, this has often involved either one-off qualitative studies, surveys of levels of trust in health or surveys where trust in health is a proxy for some other variable such as social capital. Although such quantitative work on trust has been important in contributing to debates about the possible shifting levels of trust in different societies, the 'conceptual complexity' (Calnan, Rowe and Entwistle 2006, 483) of trust suggests there is first a need for qualitative work which can then inform future quantitative research—including, for example, how to read distinctions between people talking about trust as patients and people being asked about trust as members of the general public when they may not have much knowledge or experience of the health care system (Calnan, Rowe and Entwistle 2006). Trust cannot, therefore, be boiled down to a single opinion/poll measure: there is a need to explore the different dimensions qualitatively as well as quantitatively. This issue of asking the general public about health care issues, particularly specialized subjects such as DNA banks, is highlighted in Haddow and Cunningham Burley's chapter and brings to the fore again the mediating role of the media and the key question for different public(s) about how initiatives are funded and regulated.

The focus of this volume is primarily on qualitative approaches to studying trust in relation to health, in part because of this existing emphasis on *measuring* trust (Calnan and Rowe 2004) and because our interest is in the *meanings* people attach to trust, that is, in people's 'idiosyncratic' interpretations of trust (Möllering 2006, 196). Qualitative research clearly allows us to investigate these interpretations and to tease out the relationship between what people think about trust and how this affects what they then do. It allows us, in other words, to examine the 'trivia'—the 'everyday routine making and keeping of promises and commitments' that Solomon (2000, 239) argues makes and breaks trust.

In doing so, we bear in mind the fact that there might be differences between felt and enacted trust (see Rowe and Calnan 2006a, 390, for a useful checklist of high-trust/low-trust behaviours *and* attitudes). Studies such as Huby's, and Greene et al.'s, which allow for (participant) observation of health settings, as well as interviews, are useful in relation to these distinctions, though there is a need to bear in mind that apparent signs of trusting behaviour—for example, informal written rules—may be the outcome of beliefs that are not, after all, about trust. The collection is, then, a response to the call to carry out research on trust that has a 'process perspective, obtaining a rich (typically qualitative) picture of actual trust experience, understanding the embeddedness of the relationships under investigation' (Möllering 2006, 196). The embedded nature of the research accounts in this volume are important because, as Law puts it, to consider trust 'outside of the study of particular milieu' is to run 'the risk of reifying trust as a universal property.' In the context of rapid policy development, failure to understand more about the milieux on which such policies depend means desired outcomes are unlikely (Gilson 2003).

There are, of course, issues about 'reading off' trust from what people say and write, and this, as is evident in the chapters that follow, is as true when people who take part in the research use the word trust as much as when they do not. Not talking about trust, after all, may point to the extent to which it is an unacknowledged presence rather than an absence, or as Solbjør puts it, the degree to which it is 'so taken for granted that it need not be mentioned.' These interpretative problems are accentuated by our tendency to use trust and cognate terms interchangeably. As Hall (2006) notes in relation to surveys, it might be wise, where possible, to avoid using the actual term trust or its related terms so that the research is not restricted by particular understandings or definitions. Reflexivity, then, is at the heart of researching trust, regardless of the particular methods that the contributors have chosen. In other words, the researchers are not only aware of trust as something that matters or exists between them and those who agree to take part in their research, but it is a highly interpretive act for both the researched and the researcher. As Parr and Davidson cogently argue, researching trust does not involve a 'finely tuned set of inflexible tools which can faultlessly identify and isolate evidence of trust in and between different data.'

A related point to consider in researching trust is whether it matters if trust is the intended or unintended outcome of the research. With the studies in this collection, trust was rarely the explicit focus of the research from the outset; interestingly, more often than not, it emerged as an unexpected, albeit dominant finding. To some degree this gets round the problem of what is perceived as relevant being shaped by the researchers' take on trust, though, as noted, subsequent interpretations by researchers are inevitable.

A range of methods has been drawn on in this volume. These include qualitative interviews (individually or in groups); observations, textual analysis and literature reviews. The latter, as Cook and Stepanikova argue, is increasingly necessary because of the proliferation of different types of studies on health and trust—ranging from opinion essays to empirical studies—making it difficult to distinguish which particular claims are supported by empirical findings and which are more speculative in nature. The distinction between individual and group interviews is also interesting. The women's talk in Solbjør's groups, for example, is about 'what they have heard' and about jointly constructing arguments for and against trusting. Similarly, the practitioners in the group interviews in Huby's research negotiate the meanings of trust between themselves as do the 'lay' participants in Haddow and Cunningham-Burley's chapter. Does focus-group research afford particular opportunities for the discursive and negotiated nature of health decisions to come to the fore? Although we have not included an example of longitudinal research, many of the contributors also make the case for studying trust over time to capture its iterative nature and note how in their own studies, understandings of trust have evolved. This sense of process is particularly salient when health care in different countries is experienced as ever more precarious and disjointed (Robb and Greenhalgh 2006).

The framework and funding for the research studies included in the book also varies greatly. One chapter, for example, is the outcome of a public consultation exercise funded by government (Haddow and Cunningham-Burley); another involves action research funded by health authorities (Huby). This raises interesting questions not only about the role of trust within the research relationship—see, for example, Guthrie's analysis of how patients and doctors might have responded differently to the knowledge that he, too, was a physician—but also between the researcher and their wider audiences. In Huby's chapter, for example, the action research component of the project meant that the researchers worked closely with practitioners to draw out practical implications for their work, thereby becoming 'part of the process of constructing accounts' about trust. This involved teaching health practitioners about qualitative research tools that might allow the 'softer' aspects of their service to be documented and audited—including, for example, those skills—'hunches, intuition and empathy,' which Greene et al. note 'are impossible to audit.' Huby adds, however, that in a second research setting, the lack of trust between researcher and researched left her research team feeling that their interpretations were restricted. Researching trust, like research generally, then, involves relations of trust and sometimes, as Haddow and Cunningham-Burley point out, these relations extend beyond the life of the research because of the expectations raised by taking part in a study and sometimes, as Parr and Davidson note, it is we as researchers who need to make the 'leap of faith' in relation to our data.

CONCLUSION

This collection has, at heart, been concerned with exploring what could be termed 'technologies' and 'rationalities' of trust in relation to health care. Miller and Rose (1990) in the context of their work on governmentality—and inspired by Foucault—drew the distinction between governing rationalities and technologies of government. The former, they argue, are 'the moral justifications for particular ways of exercising power by diverse authorities' (1990, 175–176), whereas the latter are the 'the complex of mundane programmes, calculations, techniques, apparatuses, documents and procedures.' Mechanic (2002) makes a similar point when he defines technologies not just as 'hardware' (2002, 460) but as organizational structures and procedures. In this collection, the governing rationalities have included the philosophies of managed care, clinical governance, informed consent and citizenship. The technologies have ranged from the hardware of disease screening to specific auditing practices. In relation to the hardware, it is worth noting, however, that, for some, the reciprocal nature of trust means that we cannot talk about trust in relation to material technologies, we can only talk about it in relation to other agents. 'Machines cannot literally be "trusted." They can only be relied upon' (Solomon 2000, 235). And yet when the women in Solbjør's study talk about trusting mammograms, are they not also telling us something important about the role of material technologies in mediating or allowing trust to take place?

Although this is not the place to expand on the implications of these rationalities and technologies for how our health practices are governed, these concepts are useful for understanding the gap that can exist between policy intentions and how policies are implemented and experienced (see O'Malley, 2004, for an account of this in relation to governmentality in general). This is why a multilayered approach is important. Trust between professionals, as we argued in previous work, may become more, not less, relevant in 'audit' cultures as professionals find themselves routinely challenged in ways that reinforce the regulatory mechanisms (Brownlie and Howson 2006). What happens when practitioners stop trusting the governing rationalities? Or when, like the practitioners in Greene et al.'s and Huby's studies, there is a 'weariness' about the cyclical nature of such rationalities? Research suggests that health professionals still rely on informal relations and local ways of doing things (Goddard and Mannion 1998), and the contributors to this volume do discuss the persistent relevance of trust in local settings.

This collection, through its focus on rationalities and technologies of trust across a range of settings, has attempted to address several key under-researched areas: how trust changes over time; how trust relates to health outcomes; trust in institutions and in the context of organisational change; trust between practitioners and the relationship between interpersonal and institutional trust. This last area has been particularly to the fore in this collection: the way trust rebounds back and forth between the inter-personal, institutional and social levels over time, shaping and reshaping these relationships.

These chapters are rich accounts of the socially embedded nature of trust, and our hope is that the collection will contribute to what is best seen as an ongoing debate about how to study trust empirically. It perhaps needs to be said, though, that many of the difficulties readers might have experienced when researching or thinking about trust, are more likely to be reflected than resolved in this book. Perhaps this in itself, however, is a statement about the nature of trust: The unavoidable complexity of life means trust can never be a 'ready made solution to a problem,' it 'is and still remains a problem' (Luhmann 1979, 30). Nevertheless, the collection hopefully offers some reassurance to researchers, new and old, about the complexities of researching in this area.

The research accounts are thick with detail, and the diversity of themes means that the collection as a whole is ambitious in scope. All contributors have wrestled with the conceptual and methodological challenges of capturing trust, but they have done so in very different settings, across different disciplines and also across different countries. The latter feature is important because of the sociocultural impact on people's beliefs about trust. Nevertheless, with the internationalization of health practices and the emergence of shared problems, not least those linked to resource rationing, it is likely that in future, sociocultural differences will remain, but similarities across countries will become, if anything, more prominent. There are risks in spreading the net so wide, but our hope, given the relative lack of empirical research in this area, is that this approach will signal the myriad ways that trust can potentially be drawn on in relation to health and, as such, help identify areas for further research.

We started this introduction by drawing attention to all the talk that there is about trust and about the danger of naming the inevitable vulnerability it involves as the elephant in the room. We end by noting Solomon's warning (2000) that there are risks, too, in *not* talking about it: not least that trust remains taken-for-granted and distrust remains something beyond our control. Researching trust, because of its inherent ambivalences, will probably always be, in equal measure, a frustrating and engaging business. Through this collection, we hope to have gone some way towards convincing readers it is also a worthwhile one.

Julie Brownlie and Alexandra Howson, July 2007

REFERENCES

Bijlsma-Frankema, K., and R. Klein Woolthuis, eds. 2005. *Trust Under Pressure: Empirical Investigations of Trust and Trust Building in Uncertain Circumstances*. Cheltenham: Edward Elgar.

Brownlie, J., and A. Howson. 2005. 'Leaps of faith' and MMR: An empirical study. *Sociology* 39 (2): 221–239.

———. 2006. 'Between the demands of truth and government': Health practitioners, trust and immunisation work. *Social Science and Medicine* 62: 433–443.

Calnan, M., and R. Rowe. 2004. *Trust in Health Care: An Agenda for Future Research*. London: The Nuffield Trust.

———. 2006. Researching trust relations in health care. Conceptual and methodological challenges—an introduction. *Journal of Health Organisation and Management* 20 (5): 349–358.

Calnan, M., R. Rowe, and V. Entwistle. 2006. Trust relations in health care: An agenda for future research. *Journal of Health Organisation and Management* 20 (5): 477–484.

Connell, N. A. D., and R. Mannion. 2006. Conceptualisations of trust in organisational literature. *Journal of Health Organisation and Management* 20 (5): 417–433.

Cook, K., R. Hardin, and M. Levi. 2005. *Cooperation without Trust*. New York: Russell Sage Foundation.

Das, T., and B. Teng. 2004. The risk based view of trust. *Journal of Business and Psychology* 19 (1): 85–116.

Entwistle, V. A., and O. Quick. 2006. Trust in the context of patient safety problems. *Journal of Health Organisation and Management* 20 (5): 397–416.

Garfinkel, H. 1967. *Studies in Ethnomethodology*. Englewood Cliffs: Prentice-Hall.

Gilson, L. 2003. Trust and the development of health care as a social institution. *Social Science & Medicine* 56 (7): 1453–1468.

———. 2006. Trust in healthcare: Theoretical perspectives and research needs. *Journal of Health Organisation and Management* 20 (5): 359–375.

Goddard, M., and R. Mannion. 1998. From competition to cooperation: New economic relationships in the National Health Service. *Health Economics* 7: 105–119.

Hall, M. A. 2006. Researching Medical Trust in the United States. *Journal of Health Organisation and Management* 20 (5): 456–467.

———. 2001. Conceptions and explanations of trust. In *Trust in Society*, ed. K. Cook. New York: Russell Sage Foundation.

———. 2002. *Trust and Trustworthiness*. New York: Russell Sage Foundation.

Illingworth, P. 2005. *Trusting Medicine: The Moral Costs of Managed Care.* New York: Routledge.
Kuhlmann, E. 2006. Traces of doubt and sources of trust. Health professions in an uncertain society. *Current Sociology* 54 (4): 607–620.
Lee-Treweek, G. 2002. Trust in complementary medicine: The case of cranial osteopathy. *The Sociological Review* 50 (1): 48–68.
Lewis, J. D., and A. Weigert. 1985. Trust as a social reality. *Social Forces* 63 (4): 967–985.
Luhmann, N. 1979. *Trust and Power.* New York: Wiley.
Mauss, M. 1993. *The Gift, The Form and Reason for Exchange in Archaic Societies.* London: Routledge.
Mechanic, D. 1998. Functions and limits of trust in providing medical care. *Journal of Health, Politics, Policy and Law* 23 (4): 661–686.
———. 2002. Socio-cultural implications of changing organizational technologies in the provision of care. *Social Science and Medicine* 54 (3): 459–467.
Miller, P., and N. Rose. 1990. Governing economic life. *Economy and Society* 19 (1): 1–27.
Möllering, G. 2005. The trust/control duality: An integrative perspective on positive expectations of others. *International Sociology* 20 (3): 283–305.
———. 2006. *Trust: Reason, Routine, Reflexivity.* Amsterdam: Elsevier.
O'Malley, P. 2004. *Risk, Uncertainty and Government.* London: Glasshouse.
O'Neill, O. 2002. *Autonomy and Trust in Bioethics.* Cambridge: Cambridge University Press.
Power, M. 1997. *The Audit Society: Rituals of Verification.* Oxford: Oxford University Press.
Putnam, R. D. 2004. Bowling together. *OECD Observer* March, 242: 14–15.
Robb, N., and T. Greenhalgh. 2006. "You have to cover up the words of the doctor." The mediation of trust in interpreted consultations in Primary Care. *Journal of Health Organisation and Management* 20 (5): 417–433.
Rowe, R., and M. Calnan. 2006a. Trust relations in health care: Developing a theoretical framework for the "new" NHS. *Journal of Health Organisation and Management* 20 (5): 376–396.
Rowe, R., and M. Calnan. 2006b. Trust relations in health care—the new agenda. *European Journal of Public Health* 16 (1): 4–6.
Shore, D. A. 2005. *The Trust Prescription for Health Care.* Chicago: Health Administration Press.
———. 2007. *The Trust Crisis in Healthcare: Causes, Consequences and Cures.* Oxford: Oxford University Press.
Simmel, G. 1950. *The Sociology of George Simmel.* New York: Free Press.
———. 1990. *The Philosophy of Money.* London: Routledge.
Solomon, R. C. 2000. Trusting. In *Heidegger, Coping and Cognitive Science*, eds. M. Wrathall and J. Malpas. Cambridge, Massachusetts: MIT Press.
Thom D. H., M. A. Hall, and L. G. Pawlson. 2004. Measuring patients' trust in physicians when assessing quality of care. *Health Affairs* 23 (4):124–132.

1 Conceptualizing Trust and Health

Julie Brownlie

1.1 INTRODUCTION

It has become common for those who write on trust to note their agreement on one thing: that trust is a difficult concept to agree on. Described, in turn, as evocative (Möllering 2006, 1), exasperating (Hollis 1998) and elusive (Gambetta 1988), some have noted a tendency to confuse causes and outcomes of trust with trust itself or to conflate trust with trustworthiness or other related terms (Hall 2006; Möllering 2006; Hardin 2002), producing what Smith graphically describes as a 'quagmire of competing interpretations' (2005, 299). Much trust research has been concerned with indicators of trustworthiness, and although trustworthiness may produce trust, to shift the focus to trustworthiness runs the risk, Möllering (2006) suggests, of reducing the trustor's[1] role to a passive one and failing to address how the *process* of trusting starts in the first place. This discussion about trust and trustworthiness, like that which follows about trust and confidence, emphasizes the extent to which there is a whole spectrum of concepts, including cooperation, reliance, familiarity, dependency, satisfaction and social capital, which are related to, but distinct from, trust (Connell and Mannion 2006). Working out these distinctions is, in practice, not easy. The contributors to this volume, like the editors, grapple empirically with the continuities and discontinuities between these concepts and in doing so are not immune from the tendencies warned of above. This chapter offers an overview of the key conceptual debates about trust and signposts how the different contributors engage with these through their research on health. In particular, it outlines different ways of theorizing the nature of trust including the relevance of the shifting relationships between interpersonal, institutional and public trust; the sociopolitical context of trust; and the relationship between trust and confidence. Three further issues are then highlighted—power, distrust and the socially differentiated nature of trust—all of which are woven through the remaining nine chapters of this volume.

1.2   THE NATURE OF TRUST

The growing body of work on trust has delineated different ways of think-ing about the bases or the nature of trust. Though this work nearly always argues for the significance of trust for our relationships and indeed for the social order, the language of trust can be contradictory. For some, trust is thought of as a concept, like power or, as we posited in the Introduction, love; for others it is an issue or a problem to be addressed. Some see it as enactment, something to be practised; others frame it as something that is allowed to happen or to unfold. This has led to a range of perspectives about the bases of trust, some more unilateral in their emphasis than others, including those which focus on: reasons (Hardin 2001); morals (Uslaner 2002); routine (Garfinkel 1967); the characteristics or dispositions of the person who trusts and is trusted (Yamagishi 2001); and emotions (Barbalet 1996). The emphasis on the affective nature of trust has been particularly foregrounded in recent commentaries on trust and health care (Brownlie and Howson 2005; Rowe and Calnan 2006; Smith 2005; though see Illing-worth [2005, 68] for a critique of Hall's [2006] argument that emotions are at the heart of the doctor–patient relationship) but also in relation to trust more generally (Barbalet 2002). In part, this could be seen as a response to those who have emphasized the cognitive dimension of trust (Hardin 2001) but, in relation to health specifically, it can also be read as a reaction to the rationalization of health care policies in high-income countries in recent years—a point returned to below.

There are also those who have attempted a more integrated understand-ing. Möllering (2006), for example, argues that although trustworthiness of actors, the taken-for-granted nature of social life and the iterative, ongoing interactions between actors—in his words, reason, reflexivity and routine—form the bases for trust, there is a missing element between these bases and trust itself: the act of suspension that allows us to make our 'leap of faith.' Möllering's argument, then, is that trust is a state of expectation which should neither be confused with the antecedents of trust nor with its actions or enactments (2006, 7). It was the difficulty of accessing these expectations *empirically*—especially when those involved may not even be conscious of them—that started two of the editors think-ing about how to retrieve trust in our own research about health (Brown-lie and Howson 2005).

This volume does not impose one understanding of the nature of trust; rather it has encouraged multiplicity. A range of perspectives, including Möllering's (2001, 2005, 2006) focus on trust as a state of expectation and Hardin's (2001) encapsulated interest model; Garfinkel's (1967) understanding of trust as a part of the taken-for-granted social order; and Mauss's (1993) and Sahlins's (1972) understanding of social soli-darity and reciprocity have been drawn on by the contributors to this collection. Across the chapters, however, there is also a strong sense of the indeterminacy of the social world, and, therefore of the need for the boundaries between these perspectives to be softened. Most obviously, this is reflected in the growing acceptance that it is almost impossible to separate out the cognitive and affective elements of trust: it is after all, as Möllering (2006) notes, rational to trust those we like. For Rowe and Calnan (2006, 390) in fact, it is the crossover between the affective and the rational that forms the basis for what they see as the new form of trust which shapes relationships between lay people and health professionals: 'informed trust.' Möllering (2006), and Luhmann (1979) both note that this more active form of trust is needed exactly because of the erosion of familiarity. The choice then, as the philosopher, Solomon (2000) has it, and as Parr and Davidson (Chapter 2) also note, cannot be the crude one between 'calculating distrust' or 'dumb but warm feelings' (233). If this were all that trust or trusting involved, we could not, as Solomon (2000) points out, make sense of the important place it has in our relationships. Moreover, the iterative nature of trust means that what might start off as a cognitive decision may, over time, evolve into something based on the affective nature of relationships (Gilson 2006). It is this evolving, trans-formative nature of trust that Solomon focuses on: trusting is not just contextual; its most exciting feature, he suggests, is that it is 'an ongoing process, a reciprocal (and not one-way) relation in which both parties as well as the relationships (and the society) are transformed through trust-ing' (2000, 234). It is trust's very nature—its anticipation of the future—that explains for Luhmann why it has a 'problematic relationship with time' (1979, 10). Not surprisingly, then, temporal issues are important for the contributors to this collection. Sheach Leith, for example, refers to her research project as an opportunity to study trust *in extremis*. Other chapters investigate trust at a time of change or flux—Huby's analysis of trust at a point of organisational change and Law's exploration of trust at a time of community crisis. This notion of 'trust under pressure' (Bijlsma-Frankema and Klein Woolthuis 2005, 2)—where people have little time or background to make their 'leap'—is interesting, especially when com-pared with studies that explore trust as part of ongoing relationships such as those between GPs and their patients (Guthrie's study in Chapter 7) or between young people and professionals in Greene et al.'s diabetes outpatient clinics (Chapter 5).

Despite the different emphases within the various perspectives noted above, trust is broadly understood to involve expectation, vulnerability and motivation (Gilson 2006). It is not strictly true to say, then, that the only thing trust researchers can agree on is the difficulty of defining trust. Most, including the contributors to this volume, accept that trust is, by its nature, linked to uncertainty (although not to risk, as this would suggest a calculability that would undermine the need for trust in the first place; Möllering 2006): 'It is generally agreed that trust becomes relevant when social interaction is based on uncertain knowledge about the likely action of another and one depends on their response for a beneficial outcome' (Smith 2005, 300). In health contexts, trust is understood to depend on expectations about the *competence* of practitioners and organisations but also to be about others acting in our *best interests* (Rowe and Calnan 2006, 377). Here again we see the importance of the cognitive and the affective. Given the role of trust in helping us to respond to indeterminacy it is not surprising that, as our consciousness of uncertainty has increased within the social sciences, usually through discourse about risk (Giddens 1991; Beck, Giddens and Lash 1994), the role and nature of trust in social practices, including health, has come under increased scrutiny. For many of the participants, both professional and lay, who took part in the research projects described, it was the managing of this uncertainty that was a key component of trust—whether in relation to the reading of mammograms; the security of DNA databanks; the nature of GP/patient relationships; expert knowledge about radiation risks; informed consent about organ retention; interagency practice; chronic illness or virtual environments.

1.2.1   Interpersonal, Institutional and Social Trust

We have, then, a working understanding of the nature of trust that takes into account contexts of uncertainty, our vulnerability in light of this and our expectation that others will be competent and act in our best interests. Following from this, a key issue in exploring the nature of trust is the relationship between interpersonal, institutional and social or generalised trust. We need to say more about this issue because it is at the heart of understanding not just trust but also health, where trust occurs at an interpersonal and at an institutional level. The latter is broadly understood to cover 'patient and public trust in clinicians and managers in general, in a particular health care organisation' and, in the United Kingdom, 'the NHS [National Health Service] as a health care system' (Rowe and Calnan 2006, 377). This definition draws on the concepts of 'public' or 'social' trust or 'generalized trust.' Gilson (2006) has suggested that trust in institutions—'institution based trust in strangers' (2006, 361)—provides a basis for generalized trust. For some, this, in turn, is defined as 'trust in random others or in social institutions without grounding in specific prior or subsequent relationships with those others' (Hardin 2001, 13). Others, however, see trust in institutions as being partly about previous experiences of them, including those shaped by media portrayals (Mechanic and Schlesinger 1996). The role of the media is a key background factor in a number of chapters, most notably Law's and Haddow and Cunningham-Burley's. Even Luhmann, who argues that 'trust and distrust depend on local milieu and personal experience,' is aware that these 'conditions may be extended by television culture' (Luhmann 2000, 103). This is clearly an area of expanding research and one that warrants further attention in relation to health.

To return, then, to the notion of social trust, in essence, the focus here is on unspecific trust or a 'generalised attitude' (Van der Schee, Groenegen and Friele 2006, 469). For those, such as Hardin (2004, 3), who have based their view of the nature of trust on people acting in specific circumstances—'A' trusts 'B' with respect to 'X'—herein lies the rub. Hardin (2001) suggests that to take seriously the notion of generalized trust, as survey questions about generally trusting other people appear to do, would mean accepting 'I trust, period, everyone, and with respect to everything' (13). Or, as Cook and Stepanikova (Chapter 10) put it, 'it is unclear who "most people" in the typical generalized trust question are.' Levi (1998, 80) has attempted to sort out the confusion by returning to the distinction between trust and trustworthiness. Only people, she argues, can be trusting, but trustworthiness can apply to individuals or institutions: when we say we trust the NHS, for example, we really mean we think its agents or employees will act in a trustworthy way.

Although we have argued for the multilayered nature of trust, we need also to be aware of these recurrent debates about the extent to which trust can be meaningfully talked of in relation to institutions or social groups. Some can accept talk of trust in institutions but struggle with the notion of trust in 'systems.' Giddens describes trust in abstract systems—the knowledge claims and regulatory patterns that underpin institutions (Smith 2005)—as does Gilson (2003), but Smith (2005) points out that the very fact that 'systems' are disembedded from local contexts and personal relations means we cannot talk about trusting them.

At a common-sense level, it is the case that when people talk about trust in the context of health, it is often unclear whether they are talking about trust in individual professionals, the medical profession, a particular organization such as a hospital, or a whole health care system such as the NHS in the United Kingdom or the Norwegian health care program. In reality, the relationships are two-way: health professionals are given a 'warrant for trust' (Misztal 1996, 121) from their association with a health profession or an organization such as a particular clinic; and, at the same time, trust in these institutions is 'built up,' almost in a symbolic interactionist sense, through the recurrent interactions between people within these settings. For Luhmann, however, whatever Weber argues, it is not easy to ascend from the micro to the macro: to 'speculate about the effects of an aggregation of individual attitudes on macro-phenomena' (2000, 105). Yet, Luhmann, too, notes that while the object of system trust is 'the system,' this only comes alive for people through the performance of experts who represent the system. Giddens (1991) represents this even more strongly when he talks about the significant role of professionals at access points to the system (Möllering 2006). In this volume, Solbjør, as we noted above, investigates the role of such experts in the abstract system of breast screening (Chapter 3), and Sheach Leith explores how parents make sense of the 'system' surrounding infant post-mortems. At the same time, as the young diabetics in Greene et al.'s study highlight, people might continue to have trust in individual professionals *despite* what they see as the limitations of the health organization or system as a whole (Entwistle and Quick 2006). There have been calls, of late, for the nature of this interplay between interpersonal and institutional trust in health settings to be empirically investigated (Calnan, Rowe and Entwistle 2006). Möllering's (2006) distinction between institutions as the bases, carriers and objects of trust is a useful way of beginning to think about how this might be done. In their case studies, both Sheach Leith and Greene et al. explore these reflexive and circular relations of trust between individuals, institutions and wider systems.

1.2.2   Shifting Patterns of Trust: The Sociopolitical Context

The empirical research on health, to date, has, for the most part, been concerned with the *amount* of trust shown at these different levels towards individual professionals, health institutions and systems. There is, for example, growing evidence suggesting that in some countries, such as the United States, trust in institutions might be in decline, even though trust in individual health professionals and in the health profession, on the whole, remains high (Hall 2006). Kuhlmann (2006) argues that European research suggests a more complex relationship between health care reorganization and trust. She notes continuing high levels of public trust in doctors in the United Kingdom (Calnan and Sanford 2004) but also that surveys in Germany, the Netherlands, England and Wales suggest that confidence in health care in general is not in decline (Van der Schee et al. 2006). Similarly, Allsop (2006, 624) notes continuing trust in doctors in the United Kingdom but a decline in trust in how they are regulated.

There is, too, a growing body of research and theorizing about *why* higher levels of trust might be placed in individual doctors rather than institutions (Calnan, Rowe and Entwistle 2006, 479). Some of this focuses on the nature of interpersonal relationships to explain why trust at this level might be more resilient, but most of it has concentrated instead on explaining the decline in public trust. The institutional performance model argues that the actual performance of institutions impacts on the public's willingness to trust (Norris 2007). Illingworth (2005), for instance, suggests that in the United States, the introduction of managed care has compromised the ability of patient/doctor relations to generate trust (37). One of the difficulties with this model, however, is that in some countries the decline in trust clearly extends well beyond medicine or health care. For some, this points to a more general erosion of social capital—the ability to sustain cooperative relations (Putnam 2000). Others suggest, however, that we also need to look to broader value changes which have undermined deference to traditional authority. In the U.K. context, Rowe and Calnan (2006, 378), for example, argue that public trust in health care has been shaped by top-down policy changes, a decline in deference towards experts and professionals *and* an erosion of social trust through breakdown of social networks. They also note the impact of the rise of consumerism, negative media coverage of the medical profession following a series of public scandals in the 1990s, and the impact of the budgetary pressures facing the NHS (see also Taylor-Gooby 2006b). The paradox here is that risk and vulnerability become sharpened and stakeholders' confidence is weakened through this very marketization of welfare societies (O'Neill 2002). This is a recurrent theme throughout this collection. Recent sociological work has also highlighted the implications of the erosion of social capital and the rise of consumerism. But it has in addition foregrounded other inter-related social changes that have consequences for social trust, including the increased concern with risk and uncertainty in neoliberal societies; processes of de-skilling in the context of increasing specialization; the disembedding of social relations that has accompanied globalization; dynamic technological changes; and the rise of the expert citizen and the 'disinformed information society' (Lash 2002, 2). In Bauman's terms, there are, as a result, fewer opportunities for 'anchoring our trust' (2001, 76).

The above suggests that it is now part of received wisdom that political and subsequent policy changes have accentuated the significance of trust in health contexts and, concomitantly, encouraged the rise of research in this area. Prior to the 1990s in the United States, for example, there was practically no medical trust research. Yet, with the introduction of managed care insurance, this research is now, to use Hall's word, 'burgeoning' (2006, 456). There is ongoing debate about the actual causes, extent and effects of such changes (O'Malley 2004), with some more optimistic than others about their implications for our ability to trust experts (Giddens 1991; Wynne 1996), but it is these changes which form the sociopolitical backdrop for some of the research stories that unfold in this collection. The wider sociopolitical context within which trust relations are played out in relation to health cannot, however, be reduced solely to concerns about risk and (dis)trust. One of the arguments of this collection is that other discourses are also evident, most notably those of altruism, reciprocity and futurism. These discourses can be linked to the idea of citizenship and to an understanding of trust as a 'public good' (see Haddow and Cunningham-Burley and Sheach Leith, this volume). Trust in these chapters is being explored at a community level, and there is a noticeable shift in language away from audit and risk to that of social morality and responsibility.

1.2.3 Conceptualizing Shifts in the Nature of Trust and Health: Trust and Confidence

Increasingly, working out what it means to trust health care institutions or health systems has involved researchers drawing on the conceptual distinction between trust and confidence. Luhmann (2000) sees both as being about expectations, but confidence carries an assumption that your expectations will not be frustrated. Trust, on the other hand, always involves choosing between options and running the risk of disappointment. Seeing confidence as dependent on the taken-for-granted nature of expert knowledge 'and social systems that control, predict or keep contingent events at bay' (Smith 2005, 307), Luhmann's definition of confidence is akin to Giddens' trust in abstract systems (Giddens 1991). For those writing about health in the United Kingdom, this distinction has been drawn on to understand recent policy changes in health care. Smith (2005) understands confidence at a system level within health care to include regulations, codes, expert knowledge and the idea of technical competence, whereas trust, which occurs at an interpersonal level, depends on cognitive but also moral and affective competence, which is inclusive of skills such as listening, sensitivity, responsiveness (Mechanic and Meyer 2000; Cook et al. 2004; see also Guthrie and Cook and Stepanikova, this volume.) Huby (Chapter 6) also makes clear the importance of such communicative skills in the context of the increasing association of quality care with team based, multidisciplinary working. Such working, as Rowe and Calnan point out, creates opportunities for trust to be 'earned through collaboration' (2006, 388) rather than, as with more traditional medical relations, defined by 'peer trust,' where authority depends on one's place in the medical hierarchy. This notion of earned trust or trust as hard 'social work' that carries obligations is also brought home in Parr and Davidson's analysis of the performativity of trust in the virtual world. Here trust is deeply relational and needs to be constantly proved through 'active listening' and the instantaneity of response across time. This is what Luhmann is getting at when he suggested that 'trust educates' (1979, 64).

Concomitantly, Smith (2005) argues that the modernization of the health service in the United Kingdom has focused on the need to improve confidence in institutional performance but, in so doing, the role of trust at the communicative level noted above has not just been neglected, it has been made redundant. Practitioners and managers are subject to surveillance and regulatory practices to ensure guidelines are followed and targets achieved. Performance indicators, and the context of 'clinical governance' in general, along with an emphasis on increased patient choice (for a good summary of trust issues in relation to patient choice, see Rowe and Calnan 2006) acts to sideline trust creating a shift from trust in professionals to confidence in a 'system of auditable rules and procedures' (Harrison and Ahmed 2002, 222). Taylor-Gooby (2006a) has framed these developments in terms of an 'efficiency' versus 'trust' dualism. Why is it, he asks, that when the NHS is more efficient it is seen as less trustworthy? Like Smith (2005), his answer is that trust is rooted in the face-to-face and emotionality rather than in economics. This 'paradox of managerialism'—that improved efficiency does not necessarily nurture trust—means we end up with a health service that meets outcomes but which 'no one likes or trusts' (Taylor-Gooby 2006b, 101). Moreover, arrangements to reduce risks carry their own risks of 'gaming behaviour' and of offering false reassurance (Rowe and Calnan 2006).

1.2.4 Moving Beyond Dualisms

Yet the relationship between trust and confidence is by no means clear (Luhmann 2000). Confidence in systems and trust in people may be different attitudes, but they are connected: the system requires trust, but the properties of the system may erode confidence and, therefore, undermine conditions for trust. Conversely, it is possible that building up trust at microlevel—for example, through belief in one's own doctor—could act to protect health care systems against loss of confidence. As already noted in the introduction, however, this remains a point for empirical investigation, not just conceptualisation.

The blurring of confidence and trust is linked to the relationship between trust and power/control, as greater control or regulation can instil confidence in systems and, thereby encourage trust in relationships within these systems. Sheach Leith (Chapter 4) engages with this relationship when exploring why parents might continue to look to legislation even though their trust in the existing law has been undermined. She argues that privileging confidence over trust can lead to 'sterile' regulations, but legislation still holds the possibility of a reinstitutionalization of trust. This reiterates a point Huby made in her discussion of accountability systems: that 'the way they are used is as, or more, important than their technicalities.' In the right conditions, Huby suggests they can 'underpin and strengthen already existing trust' even if, as Greene et al. note, practitioner involvement in such systems does not rise above 'pragmatic collusion.' Such systems, however, as Guby goes on to say, can also erode trust, and it is unlikely that by themselves they 'can engender trust where none exists in the first place.'

In the next three sections, I build on the conceptual debates outlined above, to explore three aspects that inform both the discussion so far and the chapters to follow: the interplay between trust and power; the relationship between trust and distrust; and, finally, the socially differentiated nature of trust.

1.3   TRUST AND POWER

Trust is closely or, some would argue, unavoidably, linked to the issue of power or control (Farrell 2004). For some, the issue here is one of degree: 'Modest power entails the possibility of trust, while great power asymmetry may commonly entail active distrust, and lack of power by either party blocks concern with trust altogether' (Hardin 2004, 13). Möllering, rather than focusing on levels of trust and control, prefers to think of trust and control as a duality: 'Each assume the existence of the other, refer to each other and create each other, but remain irreducible to each other' (2005, 283). The difference between the two, he suggests, turns on where we place expectations: when positive expectations are placed on structural influences, this is control, when the expectation is of 'benevolent agency' on the part of others, this is trust (Möllering 2005, 288). The point is that 'assuming the benevolence of another also assumes the particular social structures in which such benevolence is recognisable' (Möllering 2005, 290). Sheach Leith explores explicitly this relationship between control and trust in her work on organ retention, and Greene et al. and Huby, respectively, look at it in the context of teams working with older people, people with mental health problems and young people with diabetes. All these chapters serve to illustrate that even though demands for greater trust and greater control in health care might appear, at first glance, contradictory (Kuhlmann 2006), the two are inextricably connected. Power differentials have long been understood as defining of patient/physician relations; Guthrie's chapter contributes to a growing body of research that unpacks how power relations interact with the possibilities for reciprocal trust relations and, in particular, addresses the relatively unexplored area of physician trust in patients (see also Cook et al. 2004). This relationship between trust and power will become even more pertinent with the increased focus on patient choice and self-care, particularly in relation to chronic illness. How does trust fit in with increased patient empowerment? Greene et al. explore this issue in relation to young people with diabetes (Chapter 5).

This relationship between power and trust, as we have seen, is clearly at the heart of the increased focus on accountability within health care. In the United Kingdom, Rowe and Calnan (2006) have developed a model to work out the relationship between trust, accountability, power and modes of governance. They note that patient–clinician relationships have changed from trust being embodied in physicians—a paternalistic model—to an informed trust epitomised by the 'expert patient.' (Though see Guthrie, Chapter 7 for an analysis of how individual patients in practice have to work hard at maintaining their 'legitimacy' in medical encounters). As noted earlier, relationships between clinicians have changed from 'peer' to 'earned' trust, whereas clinician/manager relationships, Rowe and Calnan argue, have shifted from 'status' to 'performance' trust—from clinicians having little need to trust managers to a position now where clinicians have to work with managers to secure resources.

The chapters in this collection suggest that positing a direct inverse relationship between accountability and trust, however, might be too simplistic, as the relationship is often more nuanced with practitioners (like Greene et al.'s regulatory committee members) and 'lay people' (including the parents in Sheach Leith's chapter), often retrieving some reassurance or reward from participating in such mechanisms. Greene et al.'s finding, however, that the involvement of some staff in such committees might result in 'more regulations and paper trails for those at the coalface,' supports an argument from our earlier work, that accountability measures are invariably worked out through existing hierarchical (often gendered) divisions of labor within health care organisations (Brownlie and Howson 2006). Nevertheless, although a number of organisational risks have been associated with trusting—including high levels of trust making flexibility or change in organizations difficult—it is the possibility of power being abused which remains the key risk of trusting (Warren 1999). Discussions about the dangers or the 'dark side' of trust (Connell and Mannion 2006, 427) have been to the fore in a number of countries in recent years and in relation to health have often been debated in terms of the protection accountability measures potentially offer against such dangers. In the United Kingdom, for example, the costs of trusting are reflected in the Harold Shipman case, and in Chapter 4, Sheach Leith suggests these costs are also felt by parents caught up in cases of organ retention. Inevitably, then, we need to think not just about the nature of trust but of distrust too.

1.4   TRUST AND DISTRUST

There is considerable uncertainty, however, about how to do this. Is distrust, as Möllering (2006) queries, the absence or the opposite of trust or something different altogether? Ullmann-Margalit (2004, 61) suggests that there is trust, distrust and 'trust agnosticism,' which is the something in between which is neither trust nor distrust. After all, not trusting someone does not necessarily mean distrusting them—one may simply not have the information necessary to trust. Cook et al. (2004) have noted a need for further research on the antecedents of distrust in patient–physician relationships and have also cautioned against the assumption that the absence of trust means the presence of distrust (see also Cook and Stepanikova this volume).

For Luhmann (1979), distrust, like trust, serves a function: whereas in premodern time, trust was a strategy for reducing vulnerability, now distrust acts to reduce vulnerability and, indeed acts to create the conditions—the knowledge—necessary for trusting (Heimer 2001). Distrust, then, can become institutionalised in systems and, in the process, increase overall trust in a system. Haddow and Cunningham-Burley explore this dynamic through their analysis of the importance placed by the public(s) on the regulation of DNA databases. Solomon (2000) cogently argues that distrust is neither the opposite nor the preliminary to trust but is part of trust itself: 'The dialectic of trust and distrust is the most exciting part of the story of trust' (241). He describes 'authentic trust' as being distinct from blind or naïve trust exactly because it 'embraces distrust' (242).

Of course, distrusting carries risks too. As we have seen, the contradiction of auditing—that in addressing the problem of low trust, it potentially undermines trust—is now well documented (Power 1997). Trust and distrust are reciprocal: if someone acts as if he/she distrusts us, we are less likely to trust them in turn (see Guthrie's and Cook and Stepanikova's chapters). Distrust is, then, to use Luhmann's (1979) words 'constraining' (127). It is this worry that distrust breeds distrust that leads Braithwaite (1998) to conclude that although institutionalising distrust might make it easier to trust others interpersonally, 'distrust is best institutionalised behind the backs of actors' (369).

In the United Kingdom, talk about distrust in relation to health has been very closely tied to debates about trust/distrust in government (Brownlie and Howson 2006). Returning to the discussion about the meaning of generalized trust, the problem, is, as Hardin (2002) notes, that citizens often do not have enough information to trust government in a strong sense, though we can have more or less confidence in it. Haddow and Cunningham-Burley's chapter engages with the notion of public trust and concerns about the role of government particularly in regulating medical science (Petersen 2005). In doing so, as does Sheach Leith, they cast a critical eye over the concept of informed consent, though in their case, they do this in relation to population collections.

As Levi (1998) notes, the state is, in most cases, the most important institution for promoting public trust: 'If its information and guarantees are not credible, then the state's capacity to generate interpersonal trust will diminish' (86). This is at the heart of the argument that those who define the decline of trust in government as the problem could be missing the real issue: the decline of trustworthiness of government (Hardin 2002). As we argued in the introduction, to talk about health is unavoidably to talk about the role of the state. In earlier work, we found it useful to draw on Osborne's (1997) observation that Kant positioned medicine as a 'hybrid discipline' caught between the demands of truth and government (Brownlie and Howson 2006). We noted that where there is a perception that the government is not trustworthy, health messages, if they are to be trusted by the public, might be better 'outsourced' from government.

If we accept that trust is not necessarily by definition a good, then, as Hardin (2004) notes, this also means accepting that distrust can be benign. Distrust, such as that displayed by the community activists in Law's chapter, could, as Levi (1998) has argued, lead to improved democracy and thereby become a moral good in itself. To this extent, those who have interpreted distrust as a more active state than lack of trust might well have a point (Cook, Hardin and Levi 2005).

1.5   TRUST DIFFERENTIALS

There is a tendency, when engaging with some of these more abstract debates about trust, to forget that we do not all trust in the same way or to the same degree: trust varies according to many different factors, not least our age, gender, ethnicity and socioeconomic status. Health status is also a variable in relation to trust. To put it succinctly, the sicker and poorer you are, the less likely you are to trust (Shore 2007). Moreover, the poorer you are, the less resources you have to access the information that allows you to pursue 'active' (Giddens 1994) or 'informed' (Rowe and Calnan 2006) trust. Different patient groups also display different dynamics of trust. Just as Mechanic and Meyer (2000) noted distinctions between the accounts of patients with cancer, Lyme disease or mental health problems, so, too, do the different respondents across these chapters emphasise the importance of thinking about trust as socially differentiated. For instance, the women in Solbjør's study focus on the importance of visualizing technologies, whereas for the online users in Parr and Davidson's study, it is their very invisibility that shapes the nature of trust. Although, interestingly, it is the online mental health users who draw primarily on experiential trust; the women in Solbjør's study seem, in their accounts, to reflect an apparent trend within medicine away from trusting our readings of our own bodies towards trusting new technologies of trust: trust in information (Kuhlmann 2006). Health outcomes in relation to trust have been identified as an area in need of further research in the United States (Hall 2006) not least because of the need to first work out if trust is a precondition or an outcome. Calnan and Rowe (2006) note that one of the reasons it has proved difficult to do this is the scarcity of intervention or quasi experimental studies. In their chapter on the relationship between health outcomes and trust in the U.S. context, Cook and Stepanikova begin to address this gap while also making clear the variation in outcomes between different social groups. Greene et al. also highlight this issue of social differentiation by looking at how cultural constructions about age shape trust dynamics. Studies like Law's, meanwhile, remind us that although in the social capital literature there is a tendency for trust to be presented as an unquestioning social good, closer analysis suggests issues of justice and social differentiation are also relevant here and need to be unpacked. Haddow and Cunningham-Burley, at the same time, illustrate how, when thinking about designing research, there is also a need to think about the ways different social groupings conceive of health and trust. An emphasis on social differentiation could mean, for example, accepting the argument against a 'one size fits all approach' to public engagement on health issues (Taylor-Gooby 2006c, 76).

By necessity, it has been possible to offer only a sketch of the conceptual context within which the following chapters are embedded. This context, like trust itself, can only really come alive and have meaning when explored empirically through Luhmann's 'concrete setting(s)' (2000, 103). It is to these settings that we now turn.

NOTES

1. A note about definitions is warranted here. There is considerable debate in the literature about how those who trust and those who are trusted should

30 *Julie Brownlie*

be defined (Heimer 2001, 43). In this volume, some of the contributors have used the descriptor 'trustor' for the former and 'trustee' for the latter.

Allsop, J. 2006. Regaining trust in medicine. Professional and state strategies. *Current Sociology* 54 (4): 621–636.
Barbalet, J. M. 1996. Social emotions: Confidence, trust and loyalty. *International Journal of Sociology and Social Policy* 16 (9/10): 75–96.
———. 2002. Introduction: Why emotions are crucial. In *Emotions in Sociology, ed.* J. Barbalet. Oxford: Blackwell.
Bauman, Z. 2001. *The Individualized Society.* Cambridge: Polity Press.
Beck, U., A. Giddens, and S. Lash. 1994. *Reflexive Modernisation.* Cambridge: Polity Press.
Bijlsma-Frankema, K. and R. Klein Woolthuins, eds. 2005. *Trust Under Pressure: Empirical Investigations of Trust and Trust Building in Uncertain Circumstances.* Cheltenham: Edward Elgar.
Braithwaite, J. 1998. Institutionalising distrust, enculturating trust. In *Trust and Governance,* eds. V. Braithwaite and M. Levi. New York: Russell Sage Foundation.
Brownlie, J., and A. Howson. 2005. 'Leaps of faith' and MMR: An empirical study. *Sociology* 39 (2): 221–239.
———. 2006. 'Between the demands of truth and government': Health practitioners, trust and immunisation work. *Social Science and Medicine* 62 (2): 433–443.
Calnan, M., and R. Rowe. 2004. *Trust in Health Care: An Agenda for Future Research.* The Nuffield Trust: London.
———. 2006. Trust relations in the 'new' NHS: Theoretical and methodological challenges. Working paper 14/2006 Social Contexts and Responses to Risk Network (SCARR) [online], [cited June 29th 2007]. Available from <http://www.kent.ac.uk/scarr/papers/WkPaper14(1)CalnanRowe.pdf>
Calnan, M., R. Rowe, and V. Entwistle. 2006. Trust relations in health care: An agenda for future research. *Journal of Health Organisation and Management* 20 (5): 477–484.
Calnan, M., and E. Sanford. 2004. Public trust in healthcare: The system or the doctor? *Quality and Safety in Healthcare* 13: 92–97.
Connell, N. A. D., and R. Mannion. 2006. Conceptualisations of trust in organisational literature.' *Journal of Health Organisation and Management* 20 (5): 417–433.
Cook, K. ed. 2001. *Trust in Society.* New York: Russell Sage Foundation
Cook, K., R. Hardin, and M. Levi. 2005. *Cooperation Without Trust.* New York: Russell Sage Foundation.
Cook, K. S., R. Kramer, D. H. Thom, I. Stepanikova, S. Bailey-Mollborn, and R. M. Cooper. 2004. Trust and distrust in patient–physician relationships: Perceived determinants of high and low trust relationships in managed-care settings. In *Trust and Distrust across Organizational Contexts,* eds. R. Kramer and K. S. Cook. New York, New York: Russell Sage Foundation.
Das, T., and B. Teng. 2004. The risk based view of trust. *Journal of Business and Psychology* 19 (1): 85–116.
Entwistle, V. A. and O. Quick. 2006. Trust in the context of patient safety problems. *Journal of Health Organisation and Management* 20 (5): 397–416.
Farrell, H. 2004. Trust, distrust and power. In *Distrust,* ed. R. Hardin. New York: Russell Sage Foundation.

Gambetta, D. 1988. Foreword. In *Trust. Making and Breaking Co-operative Relations,* ed. D. Gambetta. Oxford: Basil Blackwell.

Garfinkel, H. 1967. *Studies in Ethnomethodology.* Englewood Cliffs: Prentice-Hall. Paperback edition.

Giddens, A. 1991. *The Consequences of Modernity.* Cambridge: Policy Press.

———. 1994. Risk, trust and reflexivity. In *Reflexive Modernisation,* eds. U. Beck, A. Giddens, and S. Lash. Cambridge: Polity Press.

Gilson, L. 2003. Trust and the development of health care as a social institution. *Social Science & Medicine* 56 (7): 1453–1468.

———. 2006. Trust in healthcare: Theoretical perspectives and research needs. *Journal of Health Organisation and Management* 20 (5): 359–375.

Goddard, M., and R. Mannion. 1998. From competition to cooperation: New economic relationships in the National Health Service. *Health Economics* 7 (2):105–119.

Hall, M. A. 2006. Researching medical trust in the United States. *Journal of Health Organisation and Management* 20 (5): 456–467.

Hardin, R. 1998. Trust in government. In *Trust and Governance,* eds. V. Braithwaite and M. Levi. New York: Russell Sage Foundation.

———. 2001. Conceptions and explanations of trust. In *Trust in Society,* ed. K. Cook. New York: Russell Sage Foundation.

———. 2002. *Trust and Trustworthiness.* New York: Russell Sage Foundation.

———. 2004. Distrust: Manifestations and management. In *Distrust,* ed. R. Hardin. New York: Russell Sage Foundation.

Harrison, S. and I. U. Ahmad. 2000. Medical autonomy and the UK state 1975 to 2025. *Sociology* 34 (1):129–146.

Heimer, C. A. 2001. Solving the problem of trust. In *Trust in Society,* ed. K. Cook. New York: Russell Sage Foundation.

Hollis, M. 1998. *Trust without Reason.* Cambridge: Cambridge University Press.

Illingworth, P. 2005. *Trusting Medicine: The Moral Costs of Managed Care.* New York: Routledge.

Kuhlmann, E. 2006. Traces of doubt and sources of trust. Health professions in an uncertain society. *Current Sociology* 54 (4): 607–620

Lash, S. 2002. *The Critique of Information.* London: Sage.

Lee-Treweek, G. 2002. Trust in complementary medicine: The case of cranial osteopathy. *The Sociological Review* 50 (1): 48–68.

Levi, M. 1998. A state of trust. In *Trust and Governance,* eds. V. Braithwaite and M. Levi. New York: Russell Sage Foundation.

Luhmann, N. 1979. *Trust and Power.* New York: Wiley.

———. 2000. Familiarity, confidence, trust: Problems and alternatives. In *Trust: Making and Breaking Cooperative Relations.* Electronic edition. Department of Sociology, University of Oxford, chapter 6: 94–107 ed. D. Gambetta. [online] [cited June 29th 2007]. Available from https://www.nuff.ox.ac.uk/users/gambetta/gambetta_trust%20book.pdf

Mauss, M. 1993. *The Gift, the Form and Reason for Exchange in Archaic Societies.* London: Routledge.

Mechanic, D., and S. Meyer. 2000. Concepts of trust among patients with serious illness. *Social Science and Medicine* 51 (5): 657–668.

Mechanic, D., and M. Schlesinger. 1996. The impact of managed care on patients' trust in medical care and their physicians. *JAMA* 275 (21): 1693–1697.

Misztal, B. 1996. *Trust in Modern Societies. The Search for the Bases of Moral Order.* Cambridge: Polity Press.

Möllering, G. 2001. The nature of trust: From George Simmel to a theory of expectation, interpretation and suspension. *Sociology* 35 (2): 403–420.

————. 2005. The trust/control duality: An integrative perspective on positive expectations of others. *International Sociology* 20 (3): 283–305.

————. 2006. *Trust: Reason, Routine, Reflexivity.* Amsterdam: Elsevier.

Norris, P. 2007. Skeptical patients: Performance, social capital and culture. In *The Trust Crisis In Healthcare: Causes, Consequences and Cures,* ed. D. Shore. Oxford: Oxford University Press.

O'Malley, P. 2004. *Risk, Uncertainty and Government.* London: Glasshouse.

O'Neill, O. 2002. *Autonomy and Trust in Bioethics.* Cambridge: Cambridge University Press.

Osborne, T. 1997. Of health and statecraft. In *Foucault, Health and Medicine,* eds. A. P. Petersen and R. Bunton. London: Routledge.

Petersen, A. 2005. Securing our genetic health: Engendering trust in UK Biobank. *Sociology of Health and Illness* 27 (2): 271–292.

Power, M. 1997. *The Audit Society: Rituals of Verification.* Oxford: Oxford University Press.

Putnam, R. D. 2000. *Bowling Alone: The Collapse and Revival of American Community.* Toronto: Simon & Schuster.

Rowe, R., and M. Calnan. 2006. Trust relations in health care: Developing a theoretical framework for the "new" NHS. *Journal of Health Organisation and Management* 20 (5): 376–396.

Sahlins, M. 1972. *Stone Age Economy.* New York: Aldine De Gruyter.

Shore, D. A. 2005. *The Trust Prescription for Health Care.* Health Administration Press Chicago.

————. 2007. *The Trust Crisis In Healthcare: Causes, Consequences and Cures.* Oxford: Oxford University Press.

Smith, C. 2005. Understanding trust and confidence: Two paradigms and their significance for health and social care. *Journal of Applied Philosophy* 22 (3): 299–316.

Solomon, R. C. 2000. Trusting. In *Heidegger, Coping and Cognitive Science,* eds. M. Wrathall and J. Malpas. Cambridge, MA: MIT Press.

Taylor-Gooby, P. 2006a. Trust vs. efficiency. *Prospect Magazine* April: 121.

Taylor-Gooby, P. 2006b. Trust, risk and health care reform. *Health, Risk and Society* 8 (2): 97–103.

Taylor-Gooby, P. 2006c. Social divisions of trust: Scepticism and democracy in the GM nation debate? *Journal of Risk Research* 9 (1): 75–95.

Ullmann-Margalit, E. 2004. Trust, distrust, and in between. In *Distrust,* ed. R. Hardin. New York: Russell Sage Foundation.

Uslaner, E. M. 2002. *The Moral Foundations of Trust.* Cambridge: Cambridge University Press.

Van der Schee, E., P. P. Groenewegen and R. D. Friele. 2006. Public trust in health care: A performance indicator. *Journal of Health Organisation and Management* 20 (5): 468–476.

Warren, M. E. 1999. *Democracy and Trust.* Cambridge: Cambridge University Press.

Yamagishi, T. 2001. Trust as a form of social intelligence. In *Trust in Society,* ed. K. Cook. New York: Russell Sage Foundation.

2 'Virtual Trust'

Online Emotional Intimacies in Mental Health Support

Hester Parr and Joyce Davidson

2.1 INTRODUCTION

Trust has recently been characterized as 'difficult to define and so to investigate' (Goudge and Gilson 2005, 1439), and indeed, as one of *the* 'most difficult concepts to handle in empirical research' (Brownlie and Howson 2005, 234). Researchers grappling with the concept are concerned to clarify certain qualities of people we trust, our motivations for doing so, and the processes by which trust is built and negotiated—*whom* do we trust, *why* and *how?* In our own analysis of trusting relations among users of electronic support groups (ESGs), we aim to contribute to this literature from particular (vulnerable) perspectives: those of individuals who share real-world experiences of extreme social and spatial exclusion as a result of debilitating emotional and affective disorders. By exploring circulations of trust in the virtual world, we attend further to questions of location, using sociogeographical insights to interrogate the potential significance of *where* trustful relations might take place.

Drawing on extensive qualitative research in electronic locales, and published firsthand accounts of virtual health communities, this chapter foregrounds the voices of those with anxiety disorders, as well as more general mental health problems. Participants describe profound difficulties with physically situated support groups that require their bodily presence in spaces that are communicatively demanding and immediately emotionally charged. The perceived lack of protective distance can involve intolerable exposure of a kind that ESGs are felt to avoid. ESGs are, however, described as facilitative of other forms of intimacies—closeness that is emotionally, if not spatially, present. Associated experiences of friendship, proximity and trust are highly valued by participants, and these intangible affective relations may be qualitatively different than those negotiated offline. The caring others with whom therapeutic alliances are forged online may never be *seen*, but they are nonetheless *felt* to have profound impacts on users' lives and experiences of ill-health.

This chapter draws on phenomenological insights to question the many implications of these relatively new and increasingly widespread circulations of trust for emotional health in particular and for social and spatial relations more broadly conceived. It questions whether new forms of therapeutic alliances require a reconceptualization of trust or whether the many obvious benefits are somewhat tempered by the nature of virtual trust. Further, it examines the nature of emotional involvement and detachment that is possible online. Thinking through the distances and proximities that constitute trust in virtual worlds, as they are specifically configured through questions of emotional and mental health, we aim to illuminate new ways of thinking through the problems and possibilities of trustful and caring relations. We connect and contrast insights emerging from our own materials, generated from research located within social geography, with existing studies of trust from a number of disciplinary perspectives. In our research, therefore, both the social and spatial properties of emotional co-identification are brought to the fore.

2.2   TRUST, SUBJECTIVITIES AND SOCIAL SPACE

Although trust researchers differ about, for example, the social significance of specific qualities or theoretical approaches to trust, trust is invariably portrayed as a complex and risky but *necessary* part of the business of everyday life. In the act of trusting, we invest another with a degree of power over ourselves, which is open to abuse: and so trust entails risk through exposure to the possibility of its, and our, betrayal (Luhmann 1988). Nevertheless, according to an early and still influential social theorist of trust, it is 'one of the most important synthetic forces within society' (Simmel 1950, 318); 'without the general trust that people have in each other, society itself would disintegrate' (Simmel 1990, 178). Anxious suspicion, constant vigilance, social avoidance or even paralysis would, it seems, prevail without the presence of trust to smooth the workings of everyday action and interaction: 'For the most part, individuals relate to others on the assumption that people generally are who they purport to be, will act in accordance with generally understood norms of behaviour and will meet their role obligations' (Mechanic and Meyer 2000, 657).

There is some consensus among researchers about the significance of trust for social life and that the phenomenon is inadequately articulated and understood (Bijlsma-Frankema and Klein Woolthuins 2005). In part, this is due to the extent to which it is so often taken for granted. In the course of everyday life, trusting is caught up with 'active but invisible background practices' (Solomon 2001, 236). It can thus be extraordinarily tricky to capture and examine, except, that is, where less ordinary circumstances confound implicit expectations and throw trust (through its abuse or withdrawal) into immediate relief. Think, for example, of any number of recent scandals surrounding the actions of individual politicians or priests, or of multinational (say, pharmaceutical) corporations whose actions can have negative consequences for entire populations, whether socially or region-ally constituted. Identifiably clear-cut violations of trust stand out to pro-voke public expressions of outrage and prompt perceptions and widespread reports of a 'crisis of trust' in the powerful, whether driven by profit or personal motives (O'Neill 2002a). Such suspicions are 'sticky' and seep out to undermine trust in experts of all kinds and their systems (Giddens 1991). However, in less scandalous everyday interactions, without the clar-ity of insight afforded by obvious violation, renegotiations and circula-tions of trust remain difficult to actually see. Like much of the complex background that allows our lives to 'effortlessly' unfold, trust—and indeed health—appears to demand notice only when something is amiss, where the phenomenon is dysfunctional or *misplaced* (Leder 1993).

Clearly, trust matters across every social and spatial scale (Dasgupta 1998). However, concerns about its importance and elusiveness are perhaps particularly—and for all, personally—pressing in relation to public health (O'Neill 2002b). In contexts of care, the lay public is regularly expected or even required to put our health—and less often our lives—in others' (hopefully) capable hands, without the knowledge or firsthand experience that would render such actions 'sensible' (Lupton 1996). Indeed, trust only occurs when we are partially rather than fully informed and also aware of some element of risk. 'Complete knowledge or ignorance would eliminate the need for, or possibility of, trust' (Möllering 2001, 406). Recent empiri-cal investigations have shed light on operations of trust in health contexts, focusing, for example, on parental and professional talk around vaccina-tions (Brownlie and Howson 2005); trust in doctors among patients with serious illnesses (Mechanic and Meyer 2000); and public trust in practitio-ners of complementary medicine (Lee-Treweek 2002). These investigations reveal that, even where ill-informed individuals are unable to assess risk fully, they manage to avoid the paralysis that lack of trust would entail. They do so by taking the 'leap of faith' evidently so crucial for success-ful patient–practitioner (and indeed almost all meaningful) interactions (Brownlie and Howson 2005).

Though it may be argued that we need 'good reasons' to trust another (or conversely, lack of 'bad reasons' not to), what becomes clear through these and other investigations is that the process through which we 'decide' whether another is trust*worthy* is rather mysterious and logically messy, resisting easy invocation or attribution of rationale: 'The faith which trust implies also tends to resist such calculative decision-making' (Giddens 1991, 19). For Giddens, 'trust presumes the opening out of the individual to the other [. . . and] knowledge that the other is committed and harbours no basic antagonism towards oneself' (Giddens 1991, 96). However, we cannot know this for sure, and when we trust that someone with the pro-pensity to do us harm will rather act with integrity, with our best interests at heart, we are reducing or 'suspending' rather than 'eliminating' uncertainty (Möllering 2005, 296), and our reasons for doing so are not easily isolated or unpacked. What is clear, however, is that trust allows us to act in the face of uncertainty, *as if* positive outcomes were assured.

When we place our trust in another in contexts of care, there is a potential benefit in the form of anticipated therapeutic outcome (however conceived) that can partially account for our willingness to 'take the risk.' In assessing whether or not it is 'worth it' or 'wise,' we might consider more or less tangible factors, such as professional accreditation, designed to protect our interests against unscrupulous or unqualified practitioners, or reputation around, for example, technical and interpersonal competence (Mechanic and Meyer 2000). Such factors are, however, arguably less easily identified or assessed in the kinds of peer relationships that have so far eluded the attention of trust/health researchers but that characterize increasingly prevalent and evidently effective self-help groups (Davison, Pennebaker and Dickerson 2000). In such interrelational contexts, without obvious differentials in authority or expertise, on what grounds do we build trust in our peers?

Although professionals bring a 'warrant for trust' (Misztal 1996) to encounters by virtue of qualification, peers with shared or overlapping experience (such as similar diagnoses) arguably bring warrants and qualifications of a different kind, based on the supposed authority of personal experience. However, trust still requires building and phenomenological 'work' to give meaning to interpersonal exchange (Lee-Treweek 2002). In horizontal (as opposed to hierarchical) peer relations, there is give and take of trust-building activities, including sharing of information, support and advice. Research suggests that mutual exchange and disclosure is of enormous importance in such ideally equitable (and ungovernable) relationships; there is often a strongly felt need to know that we are *sharing* a risk with the other and are equally exposed to harm. In an exploration of trust in personal, intimate relationships, Giddens, for example, emphasizes its co-constitutive nature: 'To build up trust, an individual must be both trusting and trustworthy' (1991, 96), and for Solomon (2000, 235), 'trusting is the product of participation and mutual communication in relationships.' Mutuality matters, though reliability, familiarity, and predictability are also key: 'Each person should know the other's personality, and be able to rely on regularly eliciting certain sorts of desired responses from the other [. . .] What matters is that one can rely on what the other says and does' (Giddens 1991, 96).

In empirical research as in everyday life, such constitutive qualities are not easily separable or measurable: 'There is no simple formula that will capture the intricacies of such relationships' (Solomon 2000, 235). Rather, trust is an active presence and production that we 'take the measure of,' or get a feel(ing) for, over time. We do so through repeated, sometimes trivial actions and interactions: 'The very fabric of trusting is built out of such exchanges as promises, commitments, offers, and requests and the responses they receive' (Solomon 2000, 235). Trust is a gradual, contingent and dynamic achievement, a relational accomplishment by particular subjectivities in and through particular spaces. For Solomon, to get to the heart of trust as a 'phenomenon in social space' (2000, 232) and a product of, rather than medium for, social relationships, 'One must look at the *dynamics* of the relationship, not just the "structure" of one person's attitude and beliefs towards another' (Solomon 2000, 235).

Studies should include 'multi-party communal relationships' (Solomon 2000, 232) and of course attend closely to context. Trust is never produced in a vacuum, and the phenomenological experience of its place—whether virtual or real—is an important part of its study. Approaching virtual circulations of trust can, however, be particularly tricky from some theoretical perspectives, such as that of Giddens (1991). In his account the place of trust is necessarily physical in nature, as 'co-presence' and 'face-work' are crucial for its creation and maintenance. Giddens thus raises questions as to how such intimacies could possibly emerge in the absence of proximity, or where the other cannot even be seen. Is trust, we might then ask, even possible without 'touch'? (Handy 1995). Our materials suggest that trust can indeed emerge in virtual contexts and relations and so does not necessarily or always require co-present 'face-work.' However, labour of another kind is involved, as Giddens himself recognizes in describing trust as 'creative': 'The relations which sustain basic trust are "worked at" emotionally' (Giddens 1991, 41) and again, 'trust is not and cannot be taken as "given" [. . .] it has to be worked at—the trust of the other has to be won' (Giddens 1991, 96). Such active negotiations, as we will show, allow trust to be facilitated at a distance, through emotional, if not spatial, proximity and through co-identification if not co-presence.

As literature reviewed in this section suggests, we should resist the temptation to rationalize trustful behaviour, for to do so risks losing sight of what really matters about trust. Solomon, for example, writes that 'the phenomenon of trusting is often distorted as much as it is clarified when it is opened up to philosophical examination' (Solomon 2001, 232). By removing an affective force from its place in social relations and pinning it down to dissect, we strip it from sense-giving, *meaningful* context. Hence, in philosophical treatment: 'Trusting is [often] discussed as a risk to be justified instead of an existential stance in which such questions are transcended' (Solomon 2001, 232). The step back from reason does not, however, entail 'emotionalizing' the 'object' of our concern: 'The choice between trust as a set of beliefs and trust as an "affective attitude" is a bad choice indeed. It encourages us to conceive of trust either as calculating distrust or as dumb but warm feelings' (Solomon 2001, 233). Evidently, trust can be reduced to neither, and more nuanced analyses are required to make sense of embodied and mindful negotiations of trusting relations.

Investigations should thus attend closely to the character of the context at hand but should also attempt to access and re-present the perspectives and interpretations of the subjectivities engaged. As Möllering explains, 'trust research should aim to study instances of trust assuming idiosyncratic praxis and paying attention to the fine details of interpretation [. . .] the starting point is the subjective "reality" (context) as interpreted by the trustor' (Möllering 2005, 416). By focusing closely on the perspectives of participants, we hope to reveal something of 'how trust happens' (Lee-Treweek 2002) between emotionally vulnerable participants in electronic support groups. Researching trust does not involve a finely tuned set of inflexible tools that can faultlessly identify and isolate evidence of trust in and between different data (textual and audio for example). Instead, much like participants in virtual space, researchers also engage in 'leaps of faith,' attentively trusting research participants to gesture towards, relate, name and locate trustful relations through a variety of language and affective mediums. Identifying (with) others' accounts of trust and trustful relations can be difficult and is certainly subjective. However, reading and listening to accounts of previously isolated and ill lives, the significance of newly shared information and histories, daily psychological difficulties, details of medication use and emotional trauma in virtual space, for example, suggests a range of emergent trustful relations. Our research participants subtly articulate their understandings of the risks, benefits and ambiguities of these relations as we see below. In the context of mental health research and associated histories of subjugated ill voices, it is vital that these understandings are recognised and accepted as valid—not simply held as 'suspect data' in academic suspensions of trust. Such a position does not have to imply a concomitant suspension of critical judgment but rather that reading and interpreting trust between participants, researchers and data necessarily involves trust.

2.3   BUILDING EMOTIONAL INTIMACY ONLINE

As elaborated above, trust involves 'opening out' social relations (Giddens 1991, 96) and engenders new emotional exposures, proximities and concomitant challenges in the geographical constitution of emotional life, especially for the psychologically vulnerable. Key perhaps in this context is not only the building of trust(s) but the retaining of them, especially for vulnerable people who may find social relationships demanding. By focusing on communities of support on the Internet, we highlight the social and psychic complexities involved in building and participating in virtual networks for and between people with mental health problems. Building on previous research (Parr 2002; Wooten, Yellowlees and McClaren 2003), the case study materials reveal how contemporary technologies are implicated in changing the geographies of social support and cohesion for vulnerable groups, such as ill and disabled people. We are attentive here to the dynamics of virtual communality for people with mental health problems and to how these configure *particular* temporal, proximate and distanced social relations between participants in a way that demands we rethink trustful and peer self-help. Critically interpreting the trustful relationality of user-led Internet forums for people with mental health problems will articulate how and why participation in these virtual spaces involves particular kinds of community engagements, as well as allowing reflection on diverse emotional geographies (Davidson, Bondi and Smith 2005). Echoing recent commentators who have critically evaluated Internet studies (e.g., Valentine and Holloway 2002) such an aim is elaborated through an appreciation of the mutual connectedness of on- and offline worlds. Specific dimensions of Internet use are considered; the social and emotional proximities that virtual networking engenders are teased out; and whether new opportunities are arising here for trusting and supportive social citizenships is assessed.

One key impact of the Internet for health has been a 'democratization' of medical information that has empowered individual patients to understand more about particular conditions in ways potentially disruptive of traditional hierarchies in medical relationships (Parr 2002). Current and new patients—those diagnosed with particular health conditions according to biomedical authority—can research online their treatments, prognoses and care providers, amongst other things. However, the benefits of Internet technology go beyond examples of individual accumulations of 'expert' knowledge. There are now many examples of new forms of communality amongst vulnerable people in virtual space, with chat rooms, email lists and forums focused around mutual support and the sharing of information and coping strategies around particular diagnostic categories. Internet users can cross-compare experiences, medications and progress through discussion forums that effectively 'open up' biomedicine to embodied talk and situated knowledges (Wikgren 2001). Voluntary organizations acting as advocate voices and informational sources for people with illness are also contributing to this online democratization (Fox 2001) and can be particularly influential in shaping medical and other understandings of a condition or treatment (ibid., 155), as well as in facilitating 'patient talk' around such issues. The search for, finding and reading of health-related information is, of course, infused with a politics of knowledge that makes such processes confusing, risky and ambivalent, as well as empowering, for Internet users. The pharmaceutical industry may gain influence in discussion forums in covert ways, for example, and there is a risk that certain kinds of health quizzes can encourage medical consultation and even (specific) medication use (Woodlock 2005). The complicated outcomes of accessing and sharing a range of 'mental health knowledges' also have profound implications for a group already subject to psychiatric inscription, as some empirical materials below indicate.

Although the Internet democratizes health information and gives new access pathways to treatment, many lay health consumers prefer getting their information and assistance from online support communities in the form of discussion forums, which now play an important role in how members seek, receive and interpret health news (Wikgren 2001, 306). Previous research has noted that online discussion groups seem to be particularly appropriate for individuals with 'stigmatized identities' (Johnsen, Rosenvinge and Gammon 2002, 445), as help-seeking and socialization in face-to-face interactions can be associated with 'disproportionate' levels of distress (Berger et al. 2005) for members of such groups. Some have even argued that there are unique benefits for people suffering from mental disorders in this respect, with the Internet being noted for its use in crisis and suicide prevention (Kummervold et al. 2002, 63). Positive outcomes of online peer interactions have included the overcoming of feelings of alienation and isolation, reduced stress, and development of social networks (ibid., 445), although it is equally speculated that there are negative aspects to this activity, including Internet addiction and the risk of being scammed by people 'flaming' or 'grooming' (Lebow 1998; Stein 1997)[1]. Those with particular conditions, such as schizophrenia, are understood to benefit most, as these diagnostic categories are associated with forms of social withdrawal that may suit 'anonymous' and 'faceless' online help-seeking (Haker, Lauber and Rossler 2005). However, discussion forums specific to schizophrenia can be (problematically) interpreted as lacking signs of empathy and emotional relationality (ibid.). Some researchers make claims about qualitative differences in 'types' of emotional interactions between Web-based forums orientated towards particular disorders. For example, in comparing virtual eating disorder and cancer support groups, the former have been constructed as demonstrating less intimate and supportive types of interactions (Fingeld 2000). Typical of much research about online discussion forums, then, is an evaluation of emotional relationality and social impacts through cataloguing them into typologies of communication, which are then related to rather dualistic understandings of positive or negative outcomes (Johnsen et al. 2002). Reflective writings and commentaries explore more nuanced consequences both online and offline. For example, online support might encourage diverse participation in local community activities and provide opportunities for developing social skills and relations, although little is yet known about this possibility (ibid., 449). One of the key challenges here is coming 'to grips with asynchronous, text-based environments which are bereft of the sensory inputs associated with face-to-face encounters' (Johnsen et al. 2002, 448) and in which clinical, professional or user-led moderations are implicated in producing complicated social relations surrounding psychological and emotional distress.

Although discussion forums can feature elaborate exchanges relating to mental health services, treatment and medications, it is not the content and outcomes of these particular 'medicalized' encounters that are the main focus here. Rather, a more general assessment of the emotional relationality that constitutes online self- and peer-help can provide insights into diverse trustful relations. For the most part, people who access discussion forums are geographically disparate and only virtually networked into textual environments through which emotional and social 'work' assists both the (ill) self and the collective online community. In participating in this 'work,' online users with mental health problems show themselves to be competent and effective social actors, capable of engaging in tricky relations, effecting insights and boundary-work through negotiating difficult emotional proximities and ambivalent senses of trust. Although not readily witnessed by mainstream-placed communities, nor even by other nonmental health related virtual communities, interactions in these spaces can disrupt stereotypical understandings of patients with mental health problems as socially and emotionally incompetent.

Self-writing (writing about the self) on the Internet, for example, through online discussion forums, facilitates, in this case, a graphic proximity to both illness experiences and strategies of coping through textual-talk. If people access mental health forums predisposed to trust others with similar health experiences and difficulties, then the day-to-day use of forums risks a *loss* of trust as well as the possibility of sedimenting it. The key benefit of online forums—the sharing of the experience of having mental health problems—can thus be seen as a rather difficult virtue, in that it facilitates a problematic *unsettling intimacy,* raising questions about how we can 'intimately and subjectively . . . live with the others, to live as others, without ostracism' (Kristeva 1991, 2, cited in Thien 2005, 192) and without the breakdown of trust. Elaborating this concern, Thien (ibid.) questions contemporary conceptions of intimacy reliant on a knowing, disclosive, stable self that is supposed to be operative through a universalist spatial logic of close proximity. Online mental health forums provide material through which to understand more about intimacy that 'involves unstable and strange selves "as others"' and that is facilitative of a more 'flexible intimacy' constructed through 'ambivalent and elastic spatialities' (Thien 2005, 201). Indeed, Internet forums featuring graphic discussions about mental health problems might be envisioned as spaces where people 'ceaselessly confront that otherness' (Kristeva 1982, 6) constituting illness experiences, making these very troubling experiential geographies. As such, the sharing of virtually established and difficult intimacies that can be sustained through trustful social relations may have to be flexibly constituted so as to guard against the loss of trust, as well as facilitate the building of it.

2.4 MENTAL HEALTH AND TRUST
IN VIRTUAL SOCIAL SPACE

The empirical materials highlighted below are derived from an extensive online Internet user survey designed with a combination of both closed and open-ended questions and completed by seventy-eight respondents[2]. The survey was advertised on four U.K. mental health discussion forums[3], three of which were explicitly user-led.[4] Quotations from survey responses are used below and are completely anonymised except for the gender of the respondent and the forum in question. The survey was followed up by telephone interviews with five respondents; each lasted between thirty and sixty minutes and was tape recorded and transcribed. Interviews were also conducted with managers or moderators of each Web-based forum. All materials were coded and analysed. These methods were supplemented with online overt ethnography in each of the sites, including participation in various discussion threads and live chat rooms.

2.5   CO-IDENTIFICATION IN ESTABLISHING VIRTUAL TRUST

> "There is a strong link with all of us because of our phobias, and I was very nervous at first about not being able to fit in, and most new members feel the same way, but once I posted my hello, I got such nice welcoming messages back, I felt welcome from the start. People are so nice and non-judgmental, they are knowledgeable and willing to help and they made me feel a part of a group after being on the outside for so long." (female, NPS)

The majority of people who regularly use online discussion forums in relation to mental health issues experience such spaces as ones through which profound feelings of social connectivity occur and for whom trust-building work is quickly undertaken, as the quote above shows. For those who have been disabled by mental health problems in terms of restricted access to employment, friendship networks and real-space community activity, such connectivity can seem powerfully inclusionary and significantly different to feelings of offline isolation (effects also noted by other online users such as new mothers: see Madge and O'Conner, 2005):

> "I am very isolated, I do not have a group of friends or socialize, my family are not close and all live abroad, so to me the support is vital." (female, NPS)

> "Agoraphobia can be very isolating and the forums and chat rooms give me a point of contact with the outside world." (female, NPS)

Accessing daily discussions about mental health issues in which subjective experiences and emotions are validated and responded to in nonmedical and nonjudgmental ways also means that some users feel 'insiders'— trusted and trusting members—in these discursive communities. Contrasts are sometimes drawn with the 'outside world' wherein individuals may indeed feel excluded from the workings of 'the social' and may not be trusted because of their status as people with mental health problems. Virtual communities are hence established as places where trusting relations predominate, and where personal issues can be discussed in a safe and supportive environment:

> "The community I am part of has become like an extended family to me. It is a safe place for me to meet people I've 'known' online for a long time, and to meet new people too." (female, MHUK)

> "I feel like I get better support online than I do in my everyday life, because the community I am a part of is large but also very close-knit. I also have friends who I know online and in real life, and often find that we are better able to discuss certain issues as part of the [virtual] community than we are able to face-to-face." (female, MHUK)

The communality described above indicates that online connectivity can sometimes involve offline interactions, but it is still in virtual space where these relations are more fully useful for discussing difficult mental health issues. Although there are clearly dangers here about reifying the virtual, as Valentine and Holloway (2002, 308) note, online social worlds are often described as richer and even *more intimate* than offline relationships, partly because users have time to think 'how they want to represent themselves' in particular interest networks and where people seemingly trust each other enough to share intimacies that they rarely or never would share face-to-face, even with other people with mental health problems.

Despite initial wariness of forums, technical difficulties and the demands of reading and writing while on medication and feeling unwell, many users indicate that their readiness to trust online is partly related to the open sharing of intimacies about mental health problems with others. It becomes obvious that most, if not all, active participants in a forum *are* sharing rich personal details, and it is this reciprocity and revelation that is a prime vehicle for trust-building. Here, curiously, attributions of trust feature prominently in explanations as to why detailed written accounts of illness, emotions and everyday life are shared with relative strangers:

> "I think we build up trust over time with the people we come into contact with on-line when we visit sites regularly. I trust them and they trust me. They don't judge me and try to support me as much as they can." (female, MHUK)

> "I feel I belong in a few of the forums I post on. I've been part of one forum for years now and have really gotten close to some of the older members (not age wise, but the guys that have been posting for a long time). I can ask them for advice on just about anything, and get straight answers from them. They've been through a lot with me online. I've

told them a lot of stuff about me. I feel I can trust [them], and count on [them] through thick and thin." (male, nonspecified forum)

The online building of trust can take time, and may demand support through different phases of mental health problems and periods of recovery, which means that users may morph between occupying roles as predominant providers and/or receivers of virtual care.

Ethnographic research on the four forums/Web-sites featured in the study shows that mental health talk is structured formally (through moderation and organization of pages and discussion strands); is routinized (through accepted cultures of conversation and conduct); and is occasionally disrupted (through disagreements and transgressions). Featuring strongly in all discussions of illness experience—especially for new users—is an 'invitation' to trust and to be trusting of what occurs there and to be trustworthy in one's interactions there. The emphasis is, hence, on demonstrating empathy and the bases of similarities between users, which may be markedly different to what occurs in offline interactions (even in the context of mental health services):

> "Welcome. I hope you find NPS and the bulletin board helpful. I certainly have [. . .] please don't feel worried about not fitting in. We are all very different people with different problems, but you won't find a more caring bunch, that I'm sure of. I was very nervous about posting to begin with. It does get easier and you are sure to meet people suffering similar anxieties, which will make you feel less alone and fearful." (NPS, Feb 2006)

In this sense mental health forums facilitate 'identity-becoming' opportunities whereby new and existing users are inculcated into norms of telling and expression (see also comments in Madge and O'Conner [2005] concerning the 'performativity' of cyberspace). These 'telling norms' often rehearse illness histories, treatment and medication experiences and current emotional states, a discursive structure familiar to patients who may constantly be voicing themselves and their mental states to health practitioners. In this case, however, these conventional intimacies (Thien 2005) result not in medical or psychological prescription, although this can occur; rather, users (with different levels of anonymity) engage in supportive trust-making and act to legitimate feelings held by others

Yet, despite these positive assessments of virtual trustful relations there are also difficulties associated with virtual communality and the rather risky socialization that it facilitates. In terms of trustful relations amongst vulnerable people the maintaining of trust requires hard social 'work' that necessarily goes beyond the telling of open stories about the (ill) self. In particular, there are accumulated obligations about responding to the stories of others and the everyday sharing of difficult intimacies. There is, hence, a sense in which the 'performativity' of trust is still highly relational in virtual space, as trustworthy members may have to prove their trust through demonstrating their 'active listening' to or reading of the daily stories of the difficulties of others.

2.6 MANAGING 'ILL TRUST' AND THE NECESSITY OF RESPONSE

> "When I'm online I know I can express myself, reveal my innermost thoughts and feelings without fear. I can say things online that I could never say in everyday conversation." (female, MHUK)

In the four forums that feature in this study, disruptive emotions, thoughts and behaviours can make up significant amounts of the content of virtual talk and socialisation. Postings often detail current emotional states and also ask for responses, advice or solutions to difficult situations. The dense writing of disruptive thoughts and emotions exposes other online users to difficult intimacies, especially if posted from regular members of forums, because the contents of posting must be noted and addressed in ways that challenge notions of technological 'drive-by relationships' (Putnam 2000, 177). The particular temporality of e-relationships also demands a certain 'instantness' suggestive of temporal, if not spatial, proximity. The expectations of users for responses at all times of the day and night is one of the key named benefits of Internet forum use, although when responses are not immediately forthcoming this can lead to negative emotions and even erosion of trust. Gwinnell argues, for example, that 'constant checking for new email becomes part of any internet relationship. The cycle of anticipation, fantasy, anxiety, relief from anxiety and new anticipation seems to produce obsessive-compulsive behaviour patterns' (2003, 329). Although such a damning assessment of temporal e-proximities is problematic, the suggested emotional reliance on written responses is nonetheless accurate, as one participant (telephone interview, MHF) says: "I was so disappointed that I put on a posting you know and I got, I think got one reply two days later. And that has actually put me off putting on anything emotional, not getting any response." The participant here has clearly *lost* some trust in forum members in this process. That some users may also find it difficult to put others 'on hold' as a result of these feelings suggests that e-relationships carry new responsibilities and pressures for participants.

Trustful relations in which intimacies are shared via graphic writings are undoubtedly risky. Needless to say, many users find dealing with this 'profound horror' (Radin 2006, 594) challenging:

> " [. . .] it can also be dangerous. Some subjects can trigger a bad reaction in me, so I have to be careful to avoid those areas of forums sometimes." (female, MHF)

The graphic representation of subjective irrationalities in online communities fosters new kinds of proximity to difference even between people with mental health problems (Parr 2008). This uncomfortable proximity may render it difficult to respond to postings even from members with whom trust is already established. The responsibility of trustful relations may demand rapid temporal responses, which some vulnerable people may find difficult given their psychological difficulties with exposures to others' intimate struggle (see above quote). The content of the responsive posting may also prove challenging in terms of both what is said and whether it adequately demonstrates attention to detail:

> " [. . .] you feel you've, you've then got to, to say something that's supposed to help the person, but actually you've got to be so careful about what you say. I know if I'm not well, and somebody just says just two words that are wrong it just sets me off." (Participant, telephone interview, MHF)

It is easy to imagine how trust might break down for a vulnerable person waiting for responses to a sensitive posting. For some members who may not feel well enough to 'do' constant sensitive and responsive trust-work, these challenges threaten the sustainability of trust in virtual mental health forums. Hence, the assumed distance, anonymity and transience characterizing online relationships does not necessarily feature in chronic illness forums in quite the same way as elsewhere on the Web (see also Radin 2006). Occupying online forums as places to socialise, support and be supported is certainly an ambivalent endeavour, as some 'do feel part of an on-line community, but whether I feel comfortable there is still to be decided' (female, NPS). Accumulated self-writing on forums can thus be uncomfortable, distressing and even dangerous, although it also provides users with complicated opportunities through which to practise self- and social management. Some users do this through diverse acts of distancing:

> "I have had a few friends from the phobic society, but they all were more ill than me and eventually I had to break contact or be brought down by them." (male, NPS)

> "I always seem to end up giving more support than I receive—which is why I 'cut and run' quite often." (male, NPS)

> "I emailed her [another member] back and said 'look, are you alright with this kind of personal interaction?' Because I'm very wary of that, that's one thing I'm usually very careful about, with certain people, but she didn't give me the feeling that she was going to be latching on to me or anything." (Telephone interview, MHF)

In this regard management tactics include leaving forums, breaking contact, filtering or deleting messages, simply sending visual 'hugs' without in-depth replies, recommending offline medical contact and appealing to the forum moderators and/or web-site rules. In Thien's (2005, 201) terms, this suggests that 'distance and proximity can coexist and may be configured in complex ways' in emergent trustful relations. That user-led online forums provide opportunities to practise different forms of boundary maintenance with peers is potentially useful and also signals that people with mental health problems can exercise competencies in managing trust, as well as acknowledging that 'intimacy is not simply the prerequisite for well-being' (ibid., 201–202). Distancing strategies do not suggest that intimate virtual proximities are productive of new forms of exclusions within forums. The particularities of textual relations between people suffering traumatic psychological experiences mean, however, that some boundary maintenance is thought necessary to ensure the sustainability of long-term trustful support, precisely because of the (relative) intimacy of social relations here:

> "It is a place for support, friendship and care, a place to share experiences, to gain understanding. There of course are hard times for members, who struggle day to day with living, in distress and need a place like MHUK to release emotions, to vent. IT IS NOT A PLACE of professional guidance, we don't say what people should and shouldn't do regarding their care, we don't claim to know all about treatments and illnesses and think that we can cure and prevent relapses of everyone who comes here. . . . Boundaries are important, not only in the caring field as a professional, but in friendships too and overstepping those boundaries can lead to disaster. I don't want to sound blunt and uncaring, but when I first started MHUK, I was in the very position of feeling and thinking I could hold everyone together, it soon became apparent that I could not cope with doing that and so learned to 'step back' and logically try and get the best help I could for people without thinking I had somehow destroyed them in the process."
> (Moderator statement, MHUK, www.zoo.pwp.blueyonder.co.uk)

2.7 INTERPRETING VIRTUAL TRUST FOR MENTAL HEALTH

> "Coming to this forum and chat room has helped me to make friends in everyday life, because it has helped me to trust more people." (female, MHUK)

The online co-presence of people with mental health problems, together with their detailed writing about their 'art of living,' constitutes both an uncomfortable and inspiring experience. Writing the intimate self through places of daily virtual socialization entails 'elastic spatialities' (Thien 2005, 201) of proximities and distances. In the sharing of fraught psychological and illness experiences, online users demonstrate significant 'emotional literacy,' and although such terminologies are problematic, envisioning the person with serious mental health problems as technically proficient, intimately networked, emotionally nuanced, socially competent and trust-worthy challenges stigmatizing conceptualizations of the damaged, alienated and pathologised patient-subject. At the same time, members with years of experience of virtual social relations point out the disadvantages of accessing places where trustful support happens for vulnerable groups:

> "I kind of feel like people are almost, not in a conscious way but I think new people are kind of being . . . brought into, whatever you want to call it, an online community. And once they're there, you know, they're going to have no chance of kind of like escaping. It's just going to be kind, like friendship, and come and talk to us every day. I think it's very, very negative, but in a very nice way. It's people being almost too nice to each other and they're not realising that they're not actually helping each other, they're just keeping each other in the same situation." (Telephone interview, NPS)

Such benefits and disadvantages help us to reevaluate trust and to interrogate celebratory accounts of trust-building for and in specific communities. Perhaps we have to reconfigure our conceptualizations of trust in order to understand online emotional intimacy. Virtual trust may be co-constituted differently for people with mental health problems, who are painfully aware that intimacy exists *with* responsibility, and trust happens *with* risks. Such a characterization challenges accounts of the superficiality of online relationships, and asks us to reconceptualize trust(s) in this location (Turkle 1996).

In the context of ESGs, it is also singularly significant that users 'arrive' with expectations that others sharing their space will share similar interests and, especially, their concerns around overlapping experience of mental health problems. Users are thus affectively open to trust in this context, in a manner that differs markedly from attitudes towards others in 'chance' encounters in typical negotiations of (nonvirtual) everyday life. Passing the time of day with the stranger on a train, we would not expect to have much (that matters) in common and would be surprised at our sharing a 'small world' if we discovered similar interests and aims. In marked contrast, when we log on to an ESG, our expectations of encountering similarly experienced others are strong and indeed constitute a significant part of our purpose. The point is to meet others like ourselves, and we are arguably predisposed to trust in this environment in a way that is far from typical elsewhere. Further, 'the relative anonymity aspect encourages self-expression, and the relative absence of physical and nonverbal interaction cues, for example, attractiveness facilitates the formation of relationships on other, deeper bases such as shared values and beliefs' (Bargh and McKenna 2004,

586). Turning again to questions of proximity and distance, although we are never spatially close or co-present with forum users, the emerging sense of co-identification over time can clearly facilitate affective closeness. 'Identification, also referred to as relational trust and goal congruence, arises from the extent to which the trustor and trustee share a common identity, goals and values' (Chopra and Wallace 2002).

Although ESG users share much in the way of background, perhaps also hopes and fears, it is important to note that even here there are barriers to access in terms of risks that must be managed or overcome; the initial act of logging on to the Internet in itself requires a 'leap of faith.' According to Bargh and McKenna (2004), Internet users have to trust not only the anonymity of the system but that information about them will not be used in inappropriate ways or circulated among others they do not intend to interact with. Those with mental health problems may have little opportunity to experience mutual, relational trust in the course of everyday life, and use of the Internet can enable challenges to such senses of social and spatial exclusion. As we have shown, this sense of trusted inclusion does, however, entail its own very particular responsibilities and risks. Our materials reveal that the contexts within which trust(s) are embedded are crucial to their experience and understanding: 'Trust is not generalizable, but is specific to the situation at hand' (Chopra and Wallace 2002).

2.8   CONCLUSION

As Corritore and colleagues (2003) have revealed, trust research online has been limited to date. It is however clear that the increasing use of the Internet and ESGs creates a pressing need to investigate what this means for social and spatial life. Many ESGs serve vulnerable and otherwise excluded individuals, and the overrepresentation of those with health—and especially mental health—problems should be a significant source of concern for researchers. In contemporary health care contexts, many of us trust nonproximate, unseen peers more readily than 'real-life' practitioners to inform, support, and advise us. Such changes in possibilities for articulating, negotiating and experiencing trusting relations are potentially socially significant, and we urgently need to know more about the implications of this and about the risks and responsibilities that online intimacies entail. Maloney-Krichmar and Preece (2005, 219) suggest that

'Trust is especially important in health communities and essential for reciprocity to occur in an online community. For an online community to succeed, members need to have a sense of trust that they will be treated with respect and care by the community, that their problems and concerns will be heard, and that others will provide information and support for them.'

They do however acknowledge, alongside trust researchers in offline contexts, that the practicalities of studying trust are challenging, and it seems we do need to find innovative ways to attend closely to trustful phenomena as experienced and interpreted by individuals themselves (Goudge and Gilson 2005). Ethnographic approaches are, we argue, particularly appropriate for online research, allowing us 'to develop an enriched sense of the meanings of the technology and the cultures which enable it and are enabled by it' (Hine 2000, 8). There is phenomenal(ogical) work involved in trust's maintenance (Lee-Treweek 2002), and attempts to protect trust are at least as important as the ways in which it is built in ESGs, where there may be a significant 'disposition to trust' in the first place (Ridings, Gefens and Arinze 2002, 278). Cooperative information exchange in online contexts helps create a trusting environment, but the processes by which trust is maintained, and by which users attempt to avoid its betrayal and loss, are complex and difficult to access. We suggest that response and responsibility are key to investigating and understanding trustful relations online, over time. Trust emerges from repeated and timely interactions and increased familiarity over more or less extended periods. Reciprocity and reliability are crucial, and responsiveness to personal postings helps keep trust active and alive. Trust has to be earned or won and worked at, over and over again. It can however be lost, relatively quickly and once and for all. As this chapter has shown, however (and wherever), trusting take place, its phenomenology—and perhaps especially, nonphysicality—should be a focus for future study. Researchers attending closely to the processes of its circulation, negotiation and continuation can contribute positively to understandings and perhaps also experiences of emotional health, in electronic as well as offline environments.

ACKNOWLEDGMENTS

The empirical materials that form the basis of this chapter are drawn from an ESRC-funded study (RES 000-27-0043) on 'Embodied Geographies of Inclusion: Placing Difference.' Permission to use these materials was given by Blackwell Publishing in association with Parr (2008) *Mental Health and Social Space: Towards Inclusionary Geographies.*

NOTES

1. These are terms indicating a range of abusive online behaviours, including sending abusive mailings and cultivating e-friendships for inappropriate emotional or sexual gratification.
2. The empirical materials are drawn from an ESRC-funded study (RES 000-27-0043) on 'Embodied Geographies of Inclusion: Placing Difference'; see also Parr (2008).
3. The discussion forums included: 'Mental Health in the UK' (www.zoo.pwp.blueyonder.co.uk: MHUK); 'The Mental Health Foundation' (www.

mentalhealth.org.uk: MHF); 'Little Wing' (www.littlewing.org.uk: LW); and 'The National Phobics Society' (www.phobics-society.org.uk: NPS).
4. The term 'user' has a double meaning in that it refers partly to 'users of services,' indicating that three of the four mental health forums were run by ex- or present users of psychiatric services. More generally in the chapter the term 'user' refers to participation in online forums or simply 'users of the Internet.' Moderation of forums can implicate the type of talk that occurs online with imposed rules and boundaries on the nature of exchange. In the research presented here, the moderation of user-led and nonuser-led forums did not significantly affect accounts of emergent trustful relations.

REFERENCES

Bargh, J. A., and K. Y. A. McKenna. 2004. The Internet and social life. *Annual Review of Psychology* 55: 573–590.
Berger, M., T. Wagner, and L. Baker. 2005. Internet use and stigmatised illness. *Social Science and Medicine* 61 (8): 1821–1827.
Bijlsma-Frankema, K., and R. Klein Woolthuins, eds. 2005. *Trust Under Pressure: Empirical Investigations of Trust and Trust Building in Uncertain Circumstances.* Cheltenham: Edward Elgar.
Brownlie, J., and A. Howson. 2005. Leaps of faith and MMR: An empirical study of trust. *Sociology* 39 (2): 221–239.
Chopra, K., and W. A. Wallace. 2002. Trust in Electronic Environments. Proceedings of the 36th Hawaii International Conference on System Sciences.
Corritore, C., et al. 2003. Online trust: Concepts, evolving themes, a model. *International Journal of Human-Computer Studies* 58 (6): 737–758.
Dasgupta, P. 1988. Trust as a commodity. In *Trust: Making and Breaking Cooperative Relations,* ed. D. Gambetta, 49–72. Oxford: University of Oxford.
Davidson, J., L. Bondi, and M. Smith, eds. 2005. *Emotional Geographies.* Aldershot, UK: Ashgate.
Davison, K. P., J. W. Pennebaker, and S. S. Dickerson. 2000. Who talks? The social psychology of illness support groups. *American Psychologist* Feb 55 (2): 205–217.
Fingeld, D. L. 2000. Therapeutic groups online: The good, the bad and the unknown. *Issues in Mental Health Nursing* 21 (3): 241–255.
Fox, N. 2001. Use of the Internet by medical voluntary groups in the UK. *Social Science and Medicine* 52 (1): 155–156.
Giddens, A. 1991. *Modernity and Self Identity: Self and Society in the Late Modern Age.* Cambridge: Polity Press.
Goudge, J., and L. Gilson. 2005. How can trust be investigated? Drawing lessons from past experience. *Social Science and Medicine* 61 (7): 1439–1451.
Gwinnell, E. 2003. Unique Aspects of Internet relationships. In *Telepsychiatry and E-mental Health,* eds. R. Wooten, P. Yellowlees, and P. McLaren, 327–336. London: Royal Society of Medicine Press Limited.
Haker, H., C. Lauber, and W. Rossler. 2005. Internet forums: A self-help approach for individuals with schizophrenia. *Acta Psychiatrica Scandinavica* 112 (6): 474–477.
Handy, C. 1995. Trust and the virtual. *Harvard Business Review* 73 (3): 40–50.
Hine, C. 2000. *Virtual Ethnography.* London and Thousand Oaks: Sage.
Johnsen, J.-A. K., J. H. Rosenvinge, and D. Gammon. 2002. Online group interaction and mental health: An analysis of three online discussion forums. *Scandinavian Journal of Psychology* 43 (5): 445–449.

52 Hester Parr and Joyce Davidson

Kristeva, J. 1982. *Powers of Horror: An Essay on Abjection.* New York: Columbia University Press.

———. 1991. *Strangers to Ourselves.* New York and London: Harvester Wheatsheaf.

Kummervold, P., D. Gammon, S. Bergvik, J. A. Johnsen, T. Havold, and J. Rosenvinge. 2002. Social support in a wired world: Use of on-line mental health forums in Norway. *Norwegian Journal of Psychiatry* 56 (1): 59–65.

Lebow, J. 1998. Not just talk, maybe some risk: The therapeutic potentials and pitfalls of computer mediated conversation. *Journal of Marital and Family Therapy* 24 (2): 203–206.

Leder, D. 1990. *The Absent Body.* Chicago: The University of Chicago Press.

Lee-Treweek, G. 2002. Trust in complementary medicine: The case of cranial osteopathy. *The Sociological Review* 50 (1): 48–68.

Luhmann, N. 1988. Familiarity, confidence and trust problems and alternatives. In *Trust: Making and Breaking Cooperative Relations,* ed. D. Gambetta, 94–107. Oxford: University of Oxford.

Lupton, D. 1996. Your life in their hands: Trust in the medical encounter. In *Health And The Sociology Of Emotions,* eds. V. James and J. Gabe. Oxford: Blackwell Publishers Ltd.

Madge, C., and H. O'Conner. 2005. Mothers in the making? Exploring notations of liminality in hybrid cyber/space. Transactions of the Institute of British Geographers 30 (1): 83–97.

Maloney-Krichmar, D., and J. Preece. 2005. A multilevel analysis of sociability, usability, and community dynamics in an online health community. *ACM Transactions on Computer-Human Interaction* 12 (2): 201–232.

Mechanic, D., and S. Meyer. 2000. Concepts of trust among patients with serious illness. *Social Science and Medicine* 51 (5): 657–668.

Misztal, B. A. 1996. *Trust in Modern Societies: The Search for the Bases of Social Order.* Cambridge, Massachusetts: Polity Press.

Möllering, G. 2001. The nature of trust: From Georg Simmel to a theory of expectation, interpretation and suspension. *Sociology* 35 (2): 403–420.

———. 2005. The trust/control duality. An integrative perspective on positive expectations of others. *International Sociology* 20 (3): 283–305.

O'Neill, O. 2002a. *A Question of Trust.* Cambridge: Cambridge University Press.

O'Neill, O. 2002b. *Autonomy and Trust in Bioethics.* Cambridge: Cambridge University Press.

Parr, H. 2002. New body-geographies: The embodied spaces of health and illness information on the Internet. *Environment and Planning D: Society and Space* 20 (1): 73–95.

———. 2008. *Mental Health and Social Space: Towards Inclusionary Geographies?* Oxford: Blackwell.

Putnam, R. D. 2000. *Bowling Alone: The Collapse and Revival of American Community.* Toronto: Simon & Schuster.

Radin, P. 2006. "To me, it's my life": Medical communication, trust, and activism in cyberspace. *Social Science and Medicine* 62 (3): 591–601.

Ridings, C., D. Gefen, and B. Arinze. 2002. Some antecedents and effects of trust in virtual communities. *Journal of Strategic Information Systems* 11 (3–4): 271–295.

Simmel, G. 1950. *The Sociology of Georg Simmel,* trans. and ed., K. H. Wolff. New York: Free Press.

———. 1990. *The Philosophy of Money.* London: Routledge.

Solomon, R. C. 2000. Trusting. In *Heidegger, Coping and Cognitive Science,* eds. M. Wrathall and J. Malpas. Cambridge, MA: MIT Press.

Thien, D. 2005. Intimate distances: Considering questions of "us." In *Emotional Geographies,* eds. J. Davidson, L. Bondi, and M. Smith, 191–204. Aldershot: Ashgate.

Turkle, S. 1996. Virtuality and its discontents: Searching for community in cyberspace. *The American Prospect* 24: 50–57.

Valentine, G., and S. L. Holloway. 2002. Exploring children's identities and social networks in on-line and off-line worlds. *Annals of the Association of American Geographers* 92 (2): 302–319.

Wikgren, M. 2001. Health discussions on the Internet: A study of knowledge communication through citations. *Library Information Science Research* 23 (4): 305–317.

Woodlock, D. 2005. Virtual pushers: Antidepressant Internet marketing and women. *Women's Studies International Forum* 28 (4): 304–314.

3 "*You Have to Have Trust in Those Pictures*"

A Perspective on Women's Experiences of Mammography Screening

Marit Solbjør

3.1 INTRODUCTION

Breast cancer is the most frequent cancer among women in the industrialized world, and screening—systematic examination of asymptomatic populations—is increasingly a part of public health services. In Norway a screening program for breast cancer was initiated in 1996 and became nationwide in 2004 (Cancer Registry of Norway 2005). The screening program biannually invites all women aged 50 through 69 to mammography. Women receive a letter of invitation with a preset appointment for the examination. Nearly 80 percent of those invited participated during the first round of public screening, excluding women who sought mammograms through private clinics (Hofvind 2005). In part, fear of cancer, along with the old slogan "Early detection saves lives" (Lerner 2001), might have contributed to the high participation rate, because mammography screening is widely viewed as beneficial (Sætnan 1992).

But there are also sceptical voices within medicine and among the public that question whether lives are actually saved or prolonged: early diagnosis may simply mean knowing of one's cancer for a longer period. These voices also question whether all cancers diagnosed are truly cancers; whether mass mammography screening leads to overdiagnosis and overtreatment; and whether interventions may lead to increased numbers of cancers (Baines 2003; Gotzsche and Olsen 2000; Zackrisson et al. 2006). Therefore, one can ask what fosters the high participation rate in mammography screening. We live in a society dominated by expert systems and technologies that we trust to control the inevitable risks we face (Giddens 1990). Mammography screening is such a technology and expert system, designed to reduce the risk of breast cancer deaths. The high number of participants in the Norwegian screening program may be an indication of trust in mammography as a means to reduce their risk for fatal breast cancer.

Trust in social institutions, as well as in fellow citizens, is high in Norway. In the European Social Survey 2002, Norway was top of the trust rankings of European countries, together with the other Nordic states and

Switzerland. Norwegians seem to place trust in the police, in parliament and in the legal system (Listhaug 2005). When asked about trust in sources of information about modern biotechnology in 2006, 47 percent trusted public authorities, compared to 13 percent among European Union members (Nielsen 2007). It is not clear whether Norwegians also trust health authorities when given advice about preventive health examinations.

In order to explore this question, this chapter commences with theorizing trust and introducing mammography screening as an expert system and a technology. Mammography is a visualizing technology that makes it especially interesting to explore whether and how technological aspects and expertise influence participation and trust in the efficiency of the screening program. The empirical project presented in this chapter is based on focus group interviews and explores mammography technology, expertise and visualization as connected to women's trust in mammography screening.

3.2 THEORIZING TRUST

Trust as a sociological concept maps onto the everyday, intuitive usage of the word, which may be a problem if social scientists follow suppositions, rather than looking at causal accounts and explanations of trust (Hardin 2001). What makes trust a meaningful and important concept is that it shows the process by which we reach a point where our interpretations are accepted and our awareness of the unknown is suspended (Möllering 2001). In other words, trust enters the picture when rational action is insufficient—when something remains unknown. We speak of trust when there is an element of risk and uncertainty (Giddens 1990). Yet, following Möllering (2001), trust does not eclipse rational action; rather, it is a cognitive process that combines "good reasons" with an emotional dimension (Lewis and Weigert 1985). Trust is thus based on some form of knowledge which may be personal (as when we trust in a person based on our previous experiences of him or her) or impersonal or abstract (as when we trust in institutions, rules, science). Some claim that we have more trust in those with whom we have an ongoing relationship and probably act more trustworthy ourselves if the relationship is important to us (Hardin 2001). So how is it that we trust social institutions or abstract systems?

3.2.1 Trust and Expert Systems

Our modern society is complex, and personal knowledge is more difficult to attain than in a traditional society (Giddens 1990; Möllering 2001). What is needed in the complex modern society is a strategy to reduce complexity. Trust is a strategy to reduce complexity because trust means living as if certain possible outcomes will not happen (Lewis and Weigert 1985). It is a paradox that there is less personal knowledge to base trust upon

(Möllering 2001), and at the same time this very complexity requires that we exercise more trust. One can claim that this results in a more active trust in our modern society (Giddens 1990) and more deliberate leaps of faith.

At the same time, the complexity of modern society involves abstract systems that may reduce uncertainties because they guarantee that expectations can be fulfilled independent of time and space or social relations (Giddens 1990). An expert system can be defined as a technical or professional system that organizes more or less specific areas of our social and material environment (Giddens 1990). Trust in abstract expert systems must then be something other than what Hardin (2001) calls an encapsulated interest of trust, that is, trust in other individuals with whom we have relations.

Nevertheless, abstract systems, such as expert systems, and lay people meet at particular access points (Giddens 1990), where the abstract system is represented by a specific person who provides the connection between personal trust and system trust. However, the access point is a place of tension between lay scepticism and expert knowledge and is a vulnerable area of abstract systems because it involves what Giddens (1990) refers to as facework and faceless obligations and, therefore, includes both personal trust relations and trust in the abstract.

Facework is expressed and developed through personal relations and co-presence, whereas faceless obligations are developed through faith in impersonal principles that provide statistics rather than individualized results (Giddens 1990). Trust in abstract systems takes shape as faceless obligation when knowledge of that system is unknown by lay participants, yet faith in the knowledge system is maintained. Because the expert system is complex and difficult to grasp due to its abstract character, it is especially interesting to explore what reasons and knowledge make suspension and trust possible.

3.3   MAMMOGRAPHY SCREENING AS EXPERT SYSTEM

As early as the beginning of the twentieth century, physicians claimed that early detection of breast cancer was necessary for survival (Lerner 2001). The physician made treatment decisions, and, as late as the 1960s, many physicians relied more on their own clinical experience and judgement than on statistics when deciding on breast cancer diagnosis and treatment. Still, the 1960s saw the onset of mammography screening: concomitantly, randomized controlled trials provided statistical evidence of whether or not mammography had any effect on breast cancer mortality. Results from these studies vary in their degree of support for mammography screening, and they are still being debated (Alexander et al. 1999; Andersson et al. 1988; Bjurstam et al. 1997; Frisell et al. 1997; Miller et al. 2000; Miller et al. 2002; Shapiro 1977). Discussions focus on whether or not mammography has an effect on mortality (Gotzsche and Olsen

2000; Welch 2004), false positives (Brodersen 2006) and overdiagnosis (Zackrisson et al. 2006; Zahl and Maehlen 2005). Despite the ongoing discussions it seems clear that, at least for now, those in favour of mammography screening have won this health policy debate (Sætnan 1992) as screening programs have been initiated in most Western countries. It is a paradox that governments are willing to initiate extensive and expensive screening programs while there are still ongoing scientific discussions about their effect. Questions of health policy and different parties' agendas will not be further discussed here, but a question arising from this is to what extent lay participants in screening programs are aware of these discussions and uncertainties.

Mammography screening is designed to reduce mortality by detecting presymptomatic lumps and is a complex expert system involving different kinds of experts. Radiographers manage the X-ray machines; radiologists interpret images and decide who needs further examinations; and statisticians and other scientists evaluate the program's accomplishments and effects. Lay users meet the expert system when enrolled into a screening program. The invitation letter, examination and later correspondence between the system and the women can be seen as places where face-dependent trust can be developed. Yet it is unclear whether women are aware of the complexity of expert knowledge and how they interpret these complexities and possible uncertainties.

3.4 MAMMOGRAPHY—A VISUALIZING TECHNOLOGY

Mammography is not only an expert system but is also a technological artefact. Mammography was developed as an extension of X-ray technology, photographing the breast beneath the skin by placing the breast between two glass plates. The outcome of the examination is an X-ray image of the internal breast, shaded in black and white, and its goal is to detect small lumps or condensed tissue that is apparent in the image. This image is interpreted by radiologists looking for abnormalities, and a system of cancer experts are ready to intervene with women who have abnormal mammograms. The visual interpretation by the experts can therefore entail further interventions on the bodies of screening participants.

Visualizing aspects have become invaluable in diagnostics, treatment and preventive medicine. Cartwright (1995) and Blume (1992) have explored the discovery of the X-ray and its implications in the development of medicine. After Roentgen's discovery in 1895, the X-ray technique was met with excitement as a diagnostic tool (Cartwright 1995). The X-ray provided images of the skeleton but was also used to image other parts of the body. Torso X-ray screening for tuberculosis eventually became common. Cancer screening was not the issue at that time, but some had already suggested that X-rays on healthy subjects could detect unsuspected cancers

(Cartwright 1995). This logic was not immediately embraced by radiologists, as the breast was characterized as too soft, too irregular and too changeable to image clearly with X-ray technology. Today some radiologists see the visibility of breast cancer on mammograms as clinical evidence of mammography's effect (Kaufert 1996).

There are other visualizing techniques in medical practice, such as screening for cervical cancer, osteoporosis and ultrasound imaging of the foetus. Blume (1992) studied how the standardized thermometer was introduced into medical practise and shows how technology permits delegation of the diagnosis from the sole physician to a material artefact that is embedded in a larger social setting (Blume 1992). Delegation happens when a technician performs the act of examination, for instance by using the mammography machine. The machine produces a result that is apparently objective, ready to be read and interpreted by a knowledgeable professional. The process of delegation and diagnosis presents an air of objective certainty and confidence in the result for both lay and professional users, perhaps obscuring the fact that skilled readings of mammograms are also—necessarily—interpretations. Måseide (2002) found for instance that diagnostics based on X-ray images of the lung region were negotiated between radiologists, oncologists and specialists in pulmonary medicine by discussions of thorax images at diagnostic meetings.

All these techniques require expert knowledge to interpret the results (Atkinson 1995), and visualization techniques create images for expert interpretation, requiring a high degree of abstraction (Howson 2001). For instance, the bone density scan gives its outcome in both pictures and numbers, where the numerical estimate calls for a professional interpretation, adding a 'subjective' element to the 'objective' numbers (Reventlow, Hvas, and Malterud 2006). Even though we can think of pictures as persuasive proof of objective facts, the outcome of visualization of medical procedures on bodily parts is not always predictable to its lay 'users.' For instance, Howson (2001) found that patients who were given the option to watch their own cervix on a screen during cervical colposcopy did not experience this as 'getting in touch with their body.' Rather, the process defined the cervix in medicalized terms. The women in Reventlow, Hvas and Malterud's (2006) study were influenced by the bone scan and the visualization of the bones and started interpreting their bodily experiences in relation to the bone scan. Similarly, women have various responses to ultrasound images of the foetus, sometimes 'diagnosing' the foetus as healthy or not depending on what they themselves see on the screen, sometimes puzzled by the images and dependent on medical personnel's interpretations (Sætnan 2000).

The goal of screening mammography is not to diagnose breast cancer but to separate normal from abnormal mammograms (Elmore et al. 1994). What is seen on mammograms varies, even though radiologists in charge of reading the images develop a somewhat standardized perspective through their education and experience. Debates exist, however, as to the necessary number of readings to assure quality (Moss, Blanks, and Bennett 2005). Leaving aside issues of varying image quality, differences are apparent in radiologists' interpretations of visual images (Hofvind 2005); in how abnormality is perceived; and in the concern about perceived abnormalities (Elmore et al. 1994). Mammography images are not usually shown to patients, but women know they exist, yet it is unclear how women might react to such images.

3.4.1 Visual Images as Truth

One might claim that we are living in a visual culture with sight as the primary sense: medicine is no exception in privileging the visual (Cartwright 1995; Mirzoeff 2006). The imperative of objectivity and visual modes of representation link together as instruments of 'truth' in medical knowledge (Reventlow, Hvas and Malterud 2006). Visual proof may feel more trustworthy than perceptions from other senses, perhaps because it offers a way of making concrete information that is hitherto hidden or unseen. Or maybe the image is a comprehensible object as opposed to prognoses, imperceptible lesions or the contents of test tubes, all of which contain knowledge that must be interpreted and translated by the experts? Mammography images must also be interpreted by experts, but lay users may think it is easier to spot abnormalities on a picture than to interpret other medical and scientific procedures.

To explore how women participating in a mammography screening program understand mammography technology, I now turn to empirical material, which examines whether the visual culture that we live in influences how women think about mammography and their own health. What reasons do these women have for trusting or not trusting mammography? Do the women trust in mammography as an expert system—and if so, do they trust the experts they encounter personally, or the system in the abstract?

3.5 METHODOLOGY

To explore how women experience participation in a screening program for breast cancer, it was important to hear about their perspectives and interpretations in their own words. The research group invited women due to be screened to participate in focus groups to talk about mammography and breast cancer. A total of sixty-nine women met, unequally distributed in eight groups. Each group met three times: shortly before, shortly after and six months after their mammography examination. In order to conduct a prospective design, we cooperated with the Cancer Registry of Norway— the agency in charge of the organization of the screening program. This made us dependent on their procedures when choosing a time and place for the focus group meetings. The spring of 2003 provided the last opportunity to talk to first-time participants over enrolment age in mid-Norway, and we wanted to know about their experiences as first-time participants. As it turned out, this did not imply that these women had no experience of mammography. Many had already had mammography on their own initiative. However, this was their first time responding to an invitation to participate in the public mammography screening program.

Women were sorted in groups depending on age and municipality: 50–59 and 60–69 year olds were put in different groups due to the expectation that they would have different knowledge and experiences of cancer and risk factors for breast cancer. Four municipalities were selected to represent an urban–rural dimension. Recruiting participants from sparsely populated areas or small towns gave us neighbours, friends or relatives in each group. The fact that some participants knew each other became an asset for both participation and discussions in our groups, as other researchers on women's health have found (Kitzinger 1994).

Focus group interviewing is a qualitative method that allows participants to talk freely about the subject in question (Bender and Ewbank 1994; Kitzinger and Barbour 1999; Sim 1998). A group discussion is centred round an interview guide with questions preset by the researchers but where participants' discussions with each other are in focus. All interviews were tape recorded and transcribed, and analyses were based on text transcripts. Methods used for analyzing the data were categorization, condensation of the material and interpretation (Kvale 1996). The analysis in this chapter is based on the first round of focus groups. Our research group did not primarily study women's trust in particular but rather women's experiences in general. As it turned out, trust became part of what women talked about during the first focus group sessions. None of the groups were asked directly about trust; rather, it sprang from discussions about technology, medical expertise and from talking about breast cancer and screening participation among themselves and others. Some women used the word 'trust' directly; others talked about certainties and uncertainties.

The groups differed in their discussions of this subject. The eight groups had dissimilar characteristics, and their interpretations of breast cancer and mammography differed. The analyses are centred on six of these groups, as the last two groups were less concerned with questions of trust in technology and concentrated more on other issues, such as prior and recent diseases among themselves and their families. Women in these two groups did not necessarily have less trust in mammography than the other groups who were more articulate on the subject. Rather, trust in medical expertise and technology is even stronger among these women, but more difficult to grasp in an interview, as it is more implicit in how the groups talk and what they talk about. *Not* talking about something may reflect a lack of interest or awareness, but it might also suggest that a matter is so taken for granted that it need not be mentioned. It is a challenge to grasp what people themselves may not be aware of and especially the "unknowable" knowledge that makes them trust (Möllering 2001). In what follows, I therefore concentrate on the groups where bases for trust were explicitly discussed.

3.6   TRUSTING MAMMOGRAPHY—OR NOT?

Participators in the Norwegian Screening Program for Breast Cancer hope that mammography screening might help them avoid a severe cancer experience. Women know mammography's task is to find cancer, but they most of all hope for and expect to have an 'all clear' notice. Trusting mammography to find lumps if there are any and the expectation of a message with a good content are two reasons for participating in the program. As one woman put it:

> O1: Yes, I too believe it to be very positive to have those examinations with mammography. I believe so. Because if you don't find anything it will influence you afterwards in terms of [. . .] then you'll at least feel safe. And that, that is important to me.

If nothing is found at the mammogram, women feel assured that they are well, and this may affect how they think about their own health. The safety women feel, or expect to feel after having a mammography examination makes some women neglect their own breast self-examination, and this is a concern for women in the focus groups. Some of the women in the groups ask if mammography makes it unnecessary to do the self-examination. This opened a discussion in one focus group session:

> E1: So are we going to avoid doing self-examinations then . . . because we have been to mammography?

> E2: No, I don't think we should, but for those of us who aren't really good at doing the self-examination it is good help.

> E1: But should we trust mammography 100 percent? Isn't it true that there have been mistakes made there as well? Things have been overlooked [. . .]I have this idea that I'm not going to leave everything to them. I'll keep track a bit myself as well. But that is my way of thinking. It is my body.

> E1: We can't trust this 100 percent. That has been proven.

> E2: I've heard that they have been there and not found anything, and then there has been something wrong after all.

> E3: That's the way it is with most examinations.

Women who feel unsure about whether or not they do the self-examination properly are especially glad to have the mammography screening program undertake the responsibility for finding lumps. Feeling insecure in one's own ability to detect lumps makes women welcome having a technology to help them with this chore. Women's experiences of themselves as less reliable (when doing self-palpation) than professionals doing an examination (using mammography technology) may also influence their perception of which method is best. Still the importance of doing self-examinations is highlighted by some of the women. They mention women's responsibility for their own health and body, and how this responsibility must be continued also after having the mammography examination. Seeing mammography as fallible, self-examination offers a good supplement; but, on an individual level, self-examination might feel more complex and difficult than having mammography. Many women do not trust self-examinations to provide a trustworthy result. These women trust mammography to detect cancer more than they trust themselves, but they know also of the possibility that mammography might give a wrong result.

> **R1:** But . . . can it be like a false safety that . . . doesn't have to be sure that they can find it, if there is anything. That you kind of think when one has been to an examination like that, then it is . . . is it certain that it is nothing? If they say so? Is it 100% certain?
>
> **R2:** It isn't that, is it? No, not 100% certain.
>
> **R3:** You hear about cases, when it has appeared after all, don't you [. . .] You must have heard that [. . .] it has appeared anyway. They are [. . .] well, heard about it. Should be quite safe anyway [. . .] so it must be safer than not having it. [. . .]
>
> **R4:** Must be special cases that.
>
> **R3:** Yes, but I believe that is . . . because it is like that with everything. One hundred percent, that's almost impossible.

Some women worry that mammography can give a false sense of security. They know that mammography is less than 100 percent certain. The women manage the uncertainty inherent in screening, however, by, to an extent, normalizing it: everything is uncertain, and no examination can be trusted one hundred percent. There are persistent worries that they might have breast cancer without mammography detecting it, but they find comfort in the explanation that only special cases are overlooked during the screening process. These women place trust in mammography and manage to turn their discussions about distrust around, ending up at trusting again. This raises questions of what it is they trust and what it is that makes them put their doubts aside. Is it the mammography machine as a technological artefact or the medical professionals interpreting the pictures that are trusted? Scientific discussions of what one can see from the mammograms do exist. Do women know about these discussions, and do they care about them? Is it the pictures themselves that evoke lay users' trust in mammography, and if so, why?

3.7 TRUSTING THE EQUIPMENT? THE EXPERTS? THE SYSTEM?

Women in the screening program see mammography as equipment that simplifies the process of early detection. For some it feels like the only way to gain knowledge about their own state of health when it comes to breast cancer. In other words, they trust mammography more than they trust themselves as self-examiners. Understanding cancer as a sneaking and mortal disease makes it important for them to be certain of the condition of the breast even before they can feel the potential lumps themselves.

> O2: I've heard of many who have been to mammography now, or rather, know some who've been to mammography and found lumps that are in that stage [. . .] so tiny that they couldn't be felt. So I think many have been saved by it . . . that mammography.

Mammography becomes a means to find smaller lumps than the women expect to find themselves, and thereby mammography hastens cancer detection, diagnosis and treatment compared to what would have happened if the cancer had to be found without mammography technology. Indeed, women's knowledge of breast cancer and mammography also comes from the stories of others who have been saved from severe cancer, because mammography found smaller lumps than would have been detected during self-palpation. The slogan 'early detection saves lives' (Lerner 2001) not only appears to be 'common knowledge,' but women interpret stories about cancer using this knowledge to make sense of their own experiences with breast cancer screening. Understanding cancer survival as dependent on early detection makes it necessary to lean on the technology that can obtain the earliest diagnostics for breast cancer. In this way mammography becomes a mediating technology between the women and their breasts, helping women to know the inside of their body. To what do these women ascribe mammography's superiority? Why is it better at knowing their bodies than they themselves are? Is it the machine or the experts who operate it that deserves the credit?

As far as the women are concerned, two things are necessary for finding the lump when having mammography. One is how the machine works, and the other is how medical personnel interpret the pictures. Although they know both of these to be reliable, the women are not without misgivings. The mammography machine is understood by most women as safe, even though some question the radiation they receive when having the examination. What is more important to the women is whether or not the technology is constructed to cover the whole area that has a potential for breast cancer. What can be seen when using mammography technology and what is difficult to detect are both important to the women, and they question if the reason some cancers go undetected by mammography is due to the design of the equipment.

> **G1:** I find it is a small amount of the breast that goes into the machine when they take the pictures. Can it still be trusted? Those are the thoughts I get.

> **B1:** I know of a case [. . .] a woman who has been to mammography, had her green light. But afterwards she found a lump far up in the breast [. . .] Probably wasn't part of the image.

> **B2:** No, because it depends on how they do when they put the breast into the machine. They only get [. . .] They don't see the tops.

The machine is seen as neglecting certain areas of the breast, for instance, its upper parts. These women understand that the plates of the mammography machine exclude parts of the breast and view this as a defect of the technology. The knowledge about how mammography technology functions is interpreted by these women and may be a reason for distrust in mammography screening. They know of other women who have been to mammography and had a breast cancer diagnosis a short time after, even when the result of the mammography was interpreted as normal. The question is whether or not the undetected cancer should have been detected or whether it was outside the mammography image.

The other question raised by the women is how the pictures from the mammography are interpreted. Women seem to put less emphasis on this than on the technology in their talk about having doubts about mammography. There is not much discussion about the expertise of those interpreting the mammograms nor about how mammograms can be interpreted in different ways, as is well known in medical research (Elmore et al. 1994). There is still, however, a worry about whether or not a mammography examination can find every lesion of potential breast cancer. The number of examined mammograms by each professional interpreter is seen as reassuring for the sensitivity of the examination. Still some women point to the feeling of being in a busy production line and just a number in the queue.

> **B2:** But then you can say that they examine so many breasts that they should have good knowledge of it. They look and they look and they look. The more images they see, the more knowledge. But at the same time maybe it is so many and so busy that they maybe don't use enough time on each picture? So it's double edged. But obviously they might get more statistics on how many it is.

Being part of the production line for better health makes women see themselves as one of many, and they acknowledge the necessity of statistics as part of the mammography screening expert system. The discussion brings forth reflections on how the number of screened women can make the examination and its results more accurate, even if it means having less time for each specific woman participating in the screening program. So women are aware of how the screening program, with its opportunity for experts to collect statistics and develop expertise, can make interpretations more accurate, but at the same time they point out their impression of each woman as a small piece in the system. Nevertheless, their primary focus is that routinization contributes to expertise and better diagnostics.

The above discussion, then, suggests that women know that mammography screening is complex. Yet they see the mammography examination as a way to gain knowledge of a potential breast cancer as early as possible, even before they have symptoms they can notice on their own. They also know that the technology sometimes misses breast cancer. Women in this study blame missed breast cancer primarily on the design of the technology and secondly on professional interpretations of the pictures. Being part of a screening program makes women aware of being one amongst many, and this can give reasons both for and against trusting mammography to find lumps.

Women point to good reasons for both trusting and not trusting mammography screening. From the focus group data, it appears that when women discuss the technology's materiality, the organization of the program, or the expertise involved, it leads to new rounds of doubts. Yet through these discussions, the women eventually come around to a conclusion of trust in mammography after all. They interpret their knowledge and weigh up the case for and against. Dealing with questions of technology and trust in professional knowledge, however, still do not show what it is that makes women suspend their doubts and trust mammography. What then is the suspension point? Can it be the visual aspect of mammography that somehow persuades women to trust technology and expertise?

3.8   TRUSTING THE IMAGES?

The significance of the visualizing aspect of mammography for how women come to trust is apparent in the comparison of mammography with other means for finding breast cancer. For some women the possibility of finding breast cancer is dependent on a seeing technology. They are aware of three means to locate the cancer lump in the breast: self-examination, a doctor's palpation of the breast and mammography. Ranking these, mammography, because of its visualizing technology, is thought to be the most trustworthy:

V1: Really, it is only mammography that can examine it, find it. Cause if we [...] I say that I'm not so certain of myself, then maybe the doctor can do it, but then that isn't certain either. So you can't trust that either. And we are . . . the breasts are different from each other, so how can we trust it. There isn't any lump here . . . I can't find a lump, and you can't find a lump. The doctor can't find a lump . . . but then . . . I don't know what mammography is, I believe it is some sort of X-ray, and when it comes to other X-rays they usually find things . . . So I have to trust it. They take a picture and it is an X-ray; you have to have trust in those pictures.

Familiarity with X-rays used on other parts of the body indicates that these women picture for themselves how mammography works. They have seen X-ray pictures before and know the effect of seeing one's bones. This knowledge influences their views on mammography and leads women to trust mammography more than the other methods for finding breast cancer. Breast self-examination is considered difficult, and several of these women say they do not trust their own examination. Some of them trust their doctor's breast exam more than their own, but still there can be margins of error since breasts can feel different, as noted by the women in the extract above. Finding breast cancer at an early stage, then, appears to come down to understanding the visualizing mammography as a technology that eliminates the differences between breasts and differences between examiners' experiences, whether it is a medical doctor carrying out the examination or a woman doing breast self-examination. Knowledge of different means for finding breast cancer early is interpreted by the women and weighted to find the best and most trustworthy way of saving women from breast cancer. The point of suspension seems to be rooted in the belief that it is mammography that can best find breast cancer, as the only way of eliminating uncertainties is through seeing what is really beneath the breast surface. Visualization becomes the trustworthy aspect of mammography technology, the feature that helps women put their doubts aside and trust mammography to find breast cancer so early that they can be saved from a serious disease.

One can see this more clearly in the discussion of ultrasound technology as a diagnostic tool compared to mammography. In one of the groups, two women start to discuss whether mammography or ultrasound is best for detecting breast cancer.

V1: Can you find the same thing with ultrasound as with mammography?

V2: Ultrasound is a more expensive and more thorough examination.

V1: More thorough?

V2: It looks further in, you could say. But if one should start to have all women take ultrasound, like a mass examination . . . it would be very expensive.

V1: I wouldn't mind that!

Ultrasound is classified by these women as a better but more expensive examination, and, therefore, not likely to be used in a mass screening program. When arguing for the superiority of ultrasound to mammography, it is said that ultrasound can see even deeper into the breast—a feature that makes it all the more appealing for some women in the focus groups. Even though greater efficiency does not necessarily lead to higher level of trust, for some women, better visualization techniques do give a more trustworthy result. This too indicates that visualization is the final suspension point: the point where doubts, even if they are not eliminated, can be put aside or bracketed.

3.9 CONCLUSION

This chapter has examined how and why women participating in the Norwegian screening program for breast cancer place trust in mammography as a screening technology. Other aspects of women's experiences with mammography screening are discussed elsewhere (Østerlie et al., forthcoming), but here I have chosen to compare three aspects of trust in mammography: technology, expertise, and visualization. I have chosen these aspects not only because they are theoretically interesting but also because they are prominent in the data itself.

As expected from previous research, Norwegians have trust in public institutions (Listhaug 2005), and women receiving an invitation to participate in a public screening program may trust the public health service to do what is best for them. At the same time they have, as shown above, knowledge of weaknesses in the system. Trust in public services, in and of itself, cannot explain how and why women suspend their interpretations of missed cases in breast cancer diagnostics and choose to trust mammography after all. Moreover, Giddens's (1990) faceless obligations are not enough to explain why women trust mammography before entering the program and after their first examination.

One can ask whether the mammographic image is something different from other forms of "proof" evinced through medical examinations, such as tests used on blood or urine samples, measurements of bone density or ECG. All of these are techniques for obtaining objective results about the body of the patient. We cannot answer this question from our data, but one can reflect upon it as others have done (Blume 1992; Cartwright 1995; Howson 2001). What it is possible to say is that the focus group material suggests that mammography's visualizing aspect could be the last instance of persuasion. Living in a predominantly visual culture (Mirzoeff 2006) is one way of explaining why these women suspend their doubts about the machine and the experts to place trust in the mammography program. One can claim that we are more likely to be convinced by visual proof than by other senses, such as touch (necessary for self-examination or clinical palpation). The mammogram's image of the internal breast and its lumps is seen as better proof than anything else. When the trained medical professionals look at the pictures from the mammography, lay women have to trust that the experts can see what the breast is really like.

Preventive medicine gives us the message that one might be diseased without feeling ill, leaving bodily signals untrustworthy and making us dependent on medical technology (Sachs 1995). But being dependent and trusting is not necessarily the same thing and for many women, trust co-exists—indeed is necessary—because of an awareness of uncertainty.

Trusting the technology can arise from faith in the objectivity of results, because machines can be seen as more accurate than persons. But mammography does not work by itself, it requires experts to handle it and interpret the results. The delegation of diagnosis from the physician to the machine is only partial, because the radiologist still has to interpret the images (Blume 1992). Women worry about false negatives and how certain it is that every sign of cancer is found on the mammogram. Knowledge of others who have had undetected breast cancer after participating in the screening program makes women reflect on how this can happen. Failure to detect cancer make them question mammography and its interpretations. Some of the women explain false negative diagnoses and other uncertainties in terms of how the technology works, in particular that it leaves parts of the breast unexamined. Experiencing the mammography examination as an assembly line makes women reflect on whether or not it is positive for radiologists to have so many images to interpret. The women appear to be aware of the possibility of human error whether expert or not, although awareness of uncertainties about how to interpret mammograms are less present in the focus group data than in scientific debate generally (Elmore et al. 1994). Women participating in the Norwegian mammography program seem to have faith in this expert knowledge, even when acquainted with uncertainties and are, at some point, persuaded by aspects of mammography. The image is seen as visual proof of the breast beneath the skin, leading them to take the "leap of faith." Therefore, what can be seen and what is not seen is essential for the success of the screening program.

ACKNOWLEDGMENTS

The project was funded by the Norwegian Research Council. The data has been collected and analyses have been conducted by the research group Siri Forsmo, John-Arne Skolbekken, Wenche Østerlie and Marit Solbjør at the Norwegian University of Science and Technology. Ann Rudinow Sætnan participated in the analysis.

I am grateful to Ann Rudinow Sætnan, John-Arne Skolbekken, Siri Forsmo and Marvin Rausand for comments on the drafts and for advice and support. I would also like to thank Wenche Østerlie for working with us to collect and analyse the data. Thanks to The Cancer Registry of Norway and especially to Solveig Hofvind for help with the sampling process and for support in many phases of the project.

REFERENCES

Alexander, F. E., T. J. Anderson, H. K. Brown, A. P. Forrest, W. Hepburn, A. E. Kirkpatrick, B. B. Muir, R. J. Prescott, and A. Smith. 1999. 14 years of follow-up from the Edinburgh randomised trial of breast-cancer screening. *Lancet* 353 (9168): 1903–1908.

Andersson, I., K. Aspegren, L. Janzon, T. Landberg, K. Lindholm, F. Linell, O. Ljungberg, J. Ranstam, and B. Sigfusson. 1988. Mammographic screening and mortality from breast cancer: The Malmo mammographic screening trial. *British Medical Journal* 297 (6654): 943–948.

Atkinson, P. 1995. *Medical Talk and Medical Work: The Liturgy of the Clinic.* London: Sage.

Baines, C. J. 2003. Mammography screening: Are women really giving informed consent? *Journal of National Cancer Institute* 95 (20): 1508–1511.

Bender, D.E, and D. Ewbank. 1994. The focus group as a tool for health research: Issues in design and analysis. *Health transition review: The cultural, social, and behavioural determinants of health* 4 (1): 63–79.

Bjurstam, N., L. Bjorneld, S. W. Duffy, T. C. Smith, E. Cahlin, O. Eriksson, L. O. Hafstrom, H. Lingaas, J. Mattsson, S. Persson, C. M. Rudenstam, and J. Save-Soderbergh. 1997. The Gothenburg breast screening trial: First results on mortality, incidence, and mode of detection for women ages 39–49 years at randomization. *Cancer* 80 (11): 2091–2099.

Blume, S. S. 1992. *Insight and industry. On the dynamics of technological change in medicine.* Cambridge, Massachusetts: MIT Press.

Brodersen, J. 2006. *Measuring psychosocial consequences of false-positive screening results—breast cancer as an example.* Department of General Practice, University of Copenhagen.

Brownlie, J., and A. Howson. 2005. 'Leaps of faith' and MMR: An empirical study of trust. *Sociology* 39 (2): 221–239.

Cancer Registry of Norway. 2005. *Cancer in Norway 2003.* Oslo.

Cartwright, L. 1995. *Screening the Body. Tracing Medicine's Visual Culture.* Minneapolis: University of Minnesota Press.

Elmore, J. G., C. K. Wells, C. H. Lee, D. H. Howard, and A. R. Feinstein. 1994. Variability in radiologists' interpretations of mammograms. *New England Journal of Medicine* 331 (22): 1493–1499.

Frisell, J., E. Lidbrink, L. Hellstrom, and L. E. Rutqvist. 1997. Follow up after 11 years—update of mortality results in the Stockholm mammographic screening trial. *Breast Cancer Research and Treatment* 45 (3): 263–270.

Giddens, A. 1990. *The Consequences of Modernity.* Cambridge: Polity Press.

Gotzsche, P. C., and O. Olsen. 2000. Is screening for breast cancer with mammography justifiable? *Lancet* 355 (9198): 129–134.

Hardin, R. 2001. Conceptions and explanations of trust. In *Trust in Society,* ed. K. S. Cook, 3–39. New York: Russell Sage Foundation.

Hofvind, S.S.H. 2005. *The Norwegian Breast Cancer Screening Program: Selected Process Indicators and their Utilization in Epidemiological Research,* Faculty of Medicine, University of Oslo.

Howson, A. 2001. "Watching you—watching me": Visualising techniques and the cervix. *Women's Studies International Forum* 24 (1): 97–109.

Kaufert, P. A. 1996. Women and the debate over mammography: An economic, political, and moral history. In *Gender and Health. An International Perspective,* eds. C. F. Sargent and C. B. Brettell, 167–186. New Jersey: Prentice Hall.

Kitzinger, J. 1994. *The Methodology of Focus Groups: The Importance of Interaction Between Research Participants,* 103–121. Oxford: Blackwell Publishers.

Kitzinger, J., and R. S. Barbour. 1999. *Developing Focus Group Research. Politics, Theory and Practice.* London: Sage.

Kvale, S. 1996. *InterViews. An Introduction to Qualitative Research Interviewing.* Thousand Oaks, California: Sage Publications.

Lerner, B. H. 2001. *The Breast Cancer Wars. Fear, Hope, and the Pursuit of a Cure in Twentieth-Century America.* Oxford: Oxford University Press.

Lewis, J. D., and A. Weigert. 1985. Trust as a social reality. *Social Forces* 63 (4): 967–985.

Listhaug, O. 2005. Oil wealth dissatisfaction and political trust in Norway: A resource curse? *West European Politics* 28 (4): 834–851.

Måseide, P. 2002. Røntgenbiletet og den medisinske tenkinga—ein sosiologisk analyse [The X-Ray Picture and Medical Thought—A Sociological Analysis (my translation)]. In *Helsebilder. Sunnhet og sykdom i kulturelt perspektiv,* eds. K. T. Elvebakken and P. Solvang, 193–218. Bergen: Fagbokforlaget.

Miller, A. B., T. To, C. J. Baines, and C. Wall. 2000. Canadian National Breast Screening Study-2: 13 year results of a randomized trial in women aged 50–59 years. *Journal of the National Cancer Institute* 92 (18): 1490–1499.

———. 2002. The Canadian National Breast Screening Study-1: Breast cancer mortality after 11 to 16 years of follow-up. A randomized screening trial of mammography in women age 40 to 49 years. *Annals of Internal Medicine* 137 (5 Part 1): 305–312.

Mirzoeff, N. 2006. *An introduction to visual culture.* London: Routledge.

Möllering, G. 2001. The nature of trust: From Georg Simmel to a theory of expectation, interpretation and suspension. *Sociology* 35 (2): 403–420.

Moss, S. M., R. G. Blanks, and R. L. Bennett. 2005. Is radiologists' volume of mammography reading related to accuracy? A critical review of the literature. *Clinical Radiology* 60 (6): 623–626.

Nielsen, T. H. 2007. Et spørgsmål om viden? [A question of knowledge?]. *Samfunnsspeilet* 20 (1): 13–17.

Østerlie, W., Solbjør, M., Skolbekken, J. A., Hofvind, S., Sætnan, A. R., and S. Forsmo. 2008. The limits of informed choice in organized screening. Forthcoming.

Reventlow, S. D., L. Hvas, and K. Malterud. 2006. Making the invisible body visible. Bone scans, osteoporosis and women's bodily experiences. *Social Science & Medicine* 62 (11): 2720–2731.

Sachs, L. 1995. Is There a Pathology of Prevention? The Implications of Visualizing the Invisible in Screening Programs. *Culture, Medicine and Psychiatry* 19 (4): 503–525.

Sætnan, A. R. 1992. To screen or not to screen? The impact of science on two medical technology controversies. Trondheim, Norway: University of Trondheim, Centre of Technology and Society.

———. 2000. Thirteen women's narratives of pregnancy, ultrasound, and self. In *Bodies of Technology,* eds. A. R. Sætnan, N. Oudshoorn, and M. Kirejczyk, 331–354. Columbus: Ohio State University Press.

Shapiro, S. 1977. Evidence on screening for breast cancer from a randomized trial. *Cancer* 39 (6 Suppl): 2772–2782.

Sim, J. 1998. Collecting and analysing qualitative data: Issues raised by the focus group. *Journal of Advanced Nursing* 28 (2): 345–352.

Welch, H. G. 2004. *Should I Be Tested for Cancer? Maybe Not and Here's Why.* Berkeley: University of California Press.

Zackrisson, S., I. Andersson, L. Janzon, J. Manjer, and J. P. Garne. 2006. Rate of over-diagnosis of breast cancer 15 years after end of Malmo mammographic screening trial: follow-up study. *British Medical Journal* 332 (7543): 689–692.

Zahl, P. H., and J. Maehlen. 2005. Model of outcomes of screening mammography: Spontaneous regression of breast cancer may not be uncommon. *British Medical Journal* 331 (7512): 350.

4 Restoring Trust?

Trust and Informed Consent in the Aftermath of the Organ Retention Scandal

Valerie M. Sheach Leith

" . . . for someone who never saw him or us to take away a part of him and keep it somewhere on a shelf in a jar is something too hard to think about [. . .] We trusted Alder Hey with our son's life and death, that has been misused you must ensure that this type of thing never happens again." (Chief Medical Officer's National Summit 2001)

"I have always felt that to allow the post-mortem examination of your child is an amazing gesture of trust and courage from the parent. I feel that these children are temporarily in my care and deserve every respect—and a correct and careful examination from me, so that the expectations and trust of the parents are not abused [. . .]." (Independent Review Group on the Retention of Organs at Post-mortem [Scotland] 2001).

4.1 INTRODUCTION

The organ retention scandal in the United Kingdom arose in the autumn of 1999, when it became public knowledge that organs and tissues, predominately from the bodies of infants and young children, had been routinely retained after post-mortem for subsequent diagnostic, teaching, audit and research purposes. This practice caused great distress to many parents who had not been aware of what a post-mortem entailed. In the aftermath of revelations about organ retention, parents expressed two areas of concern. First, they believed that they had not given their 'informed consent,' as it is now understood, for organs and tissue to be retained. Second, a significant number were also concerned about the body wholeness of their child (Campbell and Willis 2005; Richardson 2004; Sheach Leith 2004; Sheach Leith 2007). They felt they had buried or cremated not a 'whole' body but an 'empty shell.'

The furore surrounding post-mortem practice intensified existing concerns about a crisis of trust in the medical profession (Lupton 1996). During research conducted into aspects of the organ retention scandal, this lack of trust emerged as a key concern not only of parents but also of health care professionals, professional bodies and the government (Sheach Leith 2004). The organ retention scandal, therefore, presents a unique opportunity to study trust *in extremis*. Here, I draw upon documentary data[1] produced in the wake of the organ retention scandal to explore the steps taken ostensibly to restore trust in relation to a distinct facet of health care during a period of acute flux. My aims are threefold. First, I seek to demonstrate the complexity of the trust relationships highlighted by the organ retention scandal. Second, I consider to what extent the perceived crisis in trust can be restored through a stringent application of the doctrine of informed consent, placed at the center of reforms to post-mortem practice. Third, I move beyond informed consent to highlight the significance of other discourses, namely the gift relationship and *post-mortem citizenship*. It is argued that a consideration of the wider sociopolitical context in which consent is obtained is crucial to a full understanding of the trust relationships embedded within post-mortem practice and the potential restoration of trust. I begin by outlining the background to the organ retention scandal.

4.2 THE ORGAN RETENTION SCANDAL

The death of a child is never anything less than a tragedy for the parents, their wider family and society as a whole. Such a premature death disrupts the natural order of life and strikes at the core of contemporary Western culture, which, in constructing children as innocent (Higonnet 1998) and vulnerable (Christensen 2000), privileges the protection of the young. It was this symbolically satiated body that became the focus of attention during the organ retention scandal. By not *objecting* to a post-mortem (Human Tissue Act 1961 employed the term 'lack of objection,' not 'consent'), parents were unaware that they had also been deemed to agree to the retention of organs and tissues. Either they did not know that organs and tissues were removed from their child's body at post-mortem, or if they did, understood them to be returned to the body prior to burial or cremation. Those whose child had undergone a coroner's—or in Scotland a procurator fiscal's—post-mortem, which requires no consent, were also to find that, contrary to the legal framework, organs and tissue had been retained beyond establishing the cause of death. (See Bristol Royal Infirmary Inquiry *Interim Report* [2000] for a full and detailed account of the two types of post-mortem and the regulations governing each.)

Turner argues that we inhabit 'a society in which our major political and moral problems are expressed through the conduit of the human body' (1996, 6). In this respect, the organ retention scandal foregrounds several pressing issues. These relate to questions surrounding the relationship between body and self (Burkitt 1999; Hallam, Hockey and Howarth

1999), anxieties surrounding advancements in medical science, which have the potential to disrupt the boundaries of the body (Richardson and Turner 2002) and the commodification of the body (Scheper-Hughes, and Wacquant 2002). Channelled through the infant/child body during the organ retention scandal, these concerns presented a challenge to the legitimacy of the medical profession to control the social, legal and political discourses that shape the body. Against this complex background, issues of trust become particularly salient, not only between parents and health care professionals but also in the wider context; for as Salter (2004, 1) notes, 'The politics of medicine are driven by a triangle of intersecting forces between the profession, civil society and the state.'

In response to the revelations about post-mortem practice, several major inquiries[2] were instigated across England, Wales, Northern Ireland and Scotland. Ultimately, the concept of 'informed consent' took center stage in proposals for reforms to post-mortem practice and is now argued to be the central principle[3] of the Human Tissue Act 2004 applicable in England, Wales and Northern Ireland. However, in the Human Tissue (Scotland) Act 2006 the term *authorization* rather than consent was adopted. This conceptual shift stemmed from two main arguments. First, a conviction that the term 'informed consent,' as it is legally understood, was 'inappropriate and misleading' in the context of post-mortem practice (Independent Review Group on the Retention of Organs at Post-Mortem 2001, 16). This was felt to be particularly the case in relation to parental consent for a post-mortem, where consent can only be given in respect of the child's 'best interests'—a framework difficult to apply in these circumstances (16). Second, unlike informed consent, authorization can be given with the provision of only limited information, should parents and relatives prefer this (31). Although the concept of authorization does not map directly onto that of informed consent, as both can be argued to relate to the restoration of trust, the forthcoming discussion can be read as applying to both. The finer details of any potential differences are outwith present concerns. Thus far, I have used the term 'trust' unproblematically. I now move to remedy this.

4.3   THEORIZING AND DOCUMENTING TRUST

The following analytical discussion is firmly rooted in a sociological perspective, which recognizes and takes into account the influence of wider social structures on trusting relationships (Calnan and Rowe 2005). Within that broad framework, Guido Möllering's (2001, 2005, 2006) oeuvre proves particularly fruitful for this analysis. Möllering (2006) argues that reason, routine and reflexivity form bases for trust. The first relates to the perceived trustworthiness of trustees; the second to the 'taken for granted' and stable nature of particular situations in which trust is a feature and/or where an individual's identity is defined by their role; and the third to trust as a process which is actively constituted by actors. However, Möllering (2001, 2006) maintains that though these bases may provide the grounds for trust they do not necessarily lead to trust. What is crucial for Möllering (2001, 2006) is the 'missing element' that bridges the gap between the bases of trust and trust itself. Möllering (2006, 110) conceptualises this 'missing element' as a 'leap of faith' or 'suspension,' the latter being a 'process that enables actors to deal with irreducible uncertainty and vulnerability.' Ultimately, trust is reason, routine, and reflexivity actively combined with suspension, a two-dimensional process in which the act of suspension both springs from and validates the bases of trust. Möllering (2005, 300) also draws attention to the 'complex, dynamic and contingent—interplay of trust, control and suspension' arguing that trust and control should not be conceptualized as discrete variables—as a dualism—but as a duality. It is this rich perspective on trust which informs this analysis.

The documentary data drawn upon was conceptualized as the representations and product (Prior 1997) of the spatially and temporally specific discourses utilized by parents, health care professionals, professional bodies and the state in relation to the body and its use in medical science. All parties sought to claim as legitimate particular concerns and/or identities. Analysis of the documentary data, therefore, can facilitate understanding of the ways in which trust is actively produced as a valid area of concern, and of its significance for the construction of particular identities (e.g., the meaning of parenthood) and relationships (e.g., doctor/patient). The documentary data also allows access to the relationships of power, inherent in the organ retention scandal. These power relationships were fluid and shifted across time. At the outset of the organ retention scandal, parental concerns were given considerable prominence, for example, in the Royal Liverpool Children's Inquiry Report (2001), and the medical profession was pilloried for its failure to elicit informed consent and perceived paternalistic practices. In response, the medico-scientific community vigorously defended the need for post-mortems and the retention of organs and tissues. Later, as moves to bring in new regulatory legislation progressed, the medico-scientific community reasserted its influence by canvassing successfully for amendments to be made to the Human Tissue Act 2004.

The use of documents in social research offers a range of analytical possibilities (see Prior 2003). However, in a postpositivist framework all 'readings' are inevitably partial, as the researcher adds another layer of interpretation to the intended meanings of the author. I do not claim here, therefore, to provide a definitive reading of the 'true' meaning of trust for the various parties involved in the organ retention scandal. Rather, I proffer an analysis of the documentary data which aims to make visible the complex trust relationships highlighted by the organ retention scandal and which explores the efficacy of the steps taken to address a perceived 'crisis of trust.'

4.4   A BREACH OF TRUST

The organ retention scandal foregrounds two distinctive relationships: the first between parent and child; the second between patient and health care professional. Both are traditionally perceived to be characterized by trust. Individually these relationships may be seen as trust exemplars; together, they take on a heightened significance. The trust invested in the doctor-patient relationship by parents is intensified because it is deeply connected to the trust that their child has placed in them, leading parents to articulate a sense of acute betrayal as a result of the revelations about organ and tissue retention. Breaching this trust impacts not only on the parents as individuals but also on the essence of the parent–child relationship; this as we shall see continues beyond death.

During the inquiries into the organ retention scandal the unique nature of the parent–child relationship became highly visible. The IRGROP (2001, 31) report emphasized the sanctity of family life and stressed the quasi-spiritual nature of the parent–infant bond in particular through reference to Schoeman's (1980, 8) assertion that, 'the relationship between parent and infant involves an awareness of a kind of union between people which is perhaps more suitably described in poetic-spiritual language than in analytic moral terminology. We *share ourselves* with those with whom we are intimate' (emphasis in the original). Attention was drawn to the private and intimate character of family relationships and attendant rights against potentially unwarranted interference from other parties, such as the state or medical profession (IRGROP 2001, 31). Ideally founded on trust, the parent–child relationship is also itself a source of trust. The mother/infant dyad in particular is argued by the psychologist Erikson (1963) to be vital in facilitating the formation of a *basic trust,* which shapes the infant's capacity to trust in adult life (Giddens 1991).

Trust brings responsibility, and the parents involved in the organ retention scandal were resolute in their belief that they had a responsibility to care for and protect their child that continued *beyond* the point of death (Maclean 2002). In the Royal Liverpool Children's Inquiry Report, a mother's testimony is summarised as follows:

' . . . she would have done anything and everything in her power to protect her child. That was what she was there to do even more so in death because it was only thing she could do for her child at that stage. She had put her trust in the doctors, the midwives, the clinicians, the pathologists that they would respect her child and that they would deal with her in the way one would wish to deal with a dead person. They did not, they desecrated her. She feels let down. There was only one thing she could do and that was to protect her in death and she did not do it and she has to live with that. Alexandra's parents thought they did the right thing in consenting to post-mortem examination and now they know they did not.' (Royal Liverpool Children's Report 2001, 408)

As illustrated in the quotation above, many parents expressed feelings of doubt in their own decision-making process, and spoke of a sense of guilt at having 'failed' to protect their child, reflecting Luhmann's (1988) argument that when trust is misplaced there is an internal attribution of blame. However, determining in whom, or where, parents placed their trust is not unproblematic. The health care professionals who communicated on a one-to-one basis with parents formed only one part of a larger network of individuals, including pathologists, who may or may not have been working under the jurisdiction of the coroner or procurator fiscal, at the intersection between medicine and the law. As illustrated by the opening quotation (see page 72), parents are extremely unlikely to have personal contact with the pathologist conducting the post-mortem on their child.

In the documentary data, when parents spoke of trust, they referred to doctors and other health care professionals (see quotation above) and also to the medical profession and medical institutions in general, to specific hospitals which had cared for their child (such as Alder Hey), and to the NHS as whole, or, as immediately below, a combination of these:

"What ever (sic) you do to these doctors it will not change the way parents feel about this whole mess. It will not take away the pain we have had to suffer at the hands of somebody that you think you can trust. I now feel betrayed by the NHS. I think what we want is a sincere apology/justice and for this never to happen again and somebody should take responsibility. I need to blame somebody for this interruption to my everyday life." (PQ 120 Chief Medical Officer 2001)

"I feel as if it is going to be very difficult to trust anyone in authority, e.g., hospital doctors and such like." (PQ 182 Chief Medical Officer 2001)

"I have completely lost all faith in the medical profession. I do not trust them . . . ." (PQ 35 Chief Medical Officer 2001)

In placing their trust, parents appeared to draw on both their individual relationships with health care professionals and their positive expectations of the NHS as an institution of the welfare state.[4] Möllering (2006, 73) argues that 'patients . . . develop trust (or distrust) in the medical system to a large extent through their experiences with doctors and other medical professionals, such as nurses and midwives who represent and "embody" the institutions of medicine'. However, the exact nature of the influence of interpersonal trust on institutional trust remains nebulous (Rowe and Calnan 2006). Conversely, the institution of medicine can also provide a basis for trust in those individuals who are embedded within it. As Möllering (2006,

74) notes, 'Institutions can be seen as bases, carriers and objects of trust, trust between actors can be based on institutions, trust can be institutionalized, and institutions themselves can only be effective if they are trusted.'

The impact of changes in the institutional organization of the NHS on trust relationships are considered in greater depth below. Meantime, before moving on to explore the doctor–patient relationship, I touch briefly on the contested character of the relationship between parents and doctors/clinicians in the specific context of eliciting informed consent for a post-mortem. A recent legal case, *Stevens v. Yorkhill NHS Trust and Another* (2006), arising from a claim for damages for psychiatric injury relating to the unauthorized retention of an infant's brain, considered to what extent the participants can be viewed to have entered into a traditional doctor–patient relationship with an attendant duty of care. Although in this case, the judge ruled that the existence of a doctor–patient relationship had not been proven, establishing a duty of care depends very much on the circumstances[5], for example, care of the mother of a stillborn child. However, outside a legal framework, it could reasonably be argued that, based on the familiarity of the doctor–patient relationship and the institutionalization of trust in the same, parents took for granted that doctors owed them a duty of care.

The General Medical Council argues that 'Without trust between patients and doctors, medical care is seriously compromised' (2001). (See Gilson 2003 for a discussion of the ways in which trust affects patient–provider interaction.) Like the parent/child dyad, this relationship is often also couched in quasi-spiritual terms. As Stirrat and Gill (2005, 127) note, 'The patient–doctor relationship has traditionally been seen as covenantal rather than contractual'. Emphasizing the moral and affective aspects of the relationship, such a conceptualization bears comparison with the parent and child bond. Similarly, the trust actualized in the doctor–patient relationship supports trust in other contexts. Illingworth (2002) characterizes the traditional doctor–patient relationship as 'a rare and valuable source of trust' (32) and as 'a vessel of trust' (37) that facilitates trust relationships in the wider community, contributing, in effect to a 'trust fund' (40). It is unsurprising then that the intense betrayal felt by parents in the context of the organ retention scandal spilt out into other areas of their life. Richardson (2004, 251) suggests that parents experienced multiple losses, including a loss of self-respect, a loss of respect for professionals, a loss of trust in the NHS and a loss of innocence: 'This loss [of innocence] means that natural reactions to many things are tarnished, people and things can no longer be taken at face value. For example, suspicions arise where before trust was freely given.' For parents, the doctor–patient relationship was no longer 'a vessel of trust' and the NHS no longer a trusted institution. They no longer knew in whom, or in what, to trust; perhaps they could not even trust themselves. In turn, in the aftermath of the organ retention scandal, health care professionals were bewildered that a practice they had viewed as routine had caused such uproar (Bennet 2001), and the government's invasion of medical territory was given further impetus (Salter 2004). Against this troubled background, if the doctrine of informed consent was perceived as a key step in restoring trust, the burden placed upon it was immense.

4.5   INFORMED CONSENT, TRUST, CONFIDENCE, CONTROL?

Drawing on the documentary data produced in the wake of the organ retention scandal it could be argued that there was an acknowledgement that trust had been lost; that trust was important in the effective delivery of health care; and, furthermore, that there was evidence of a wish to rebuild trust. The IRGROP (2001, 2), for example, stated that 'past practice in Scotland has . . . led to a significant breakdown in trust between relatives and the medical profession [. . .] the Group has identified a clear need for a major cultural shift if this trust is to be restored.' As the doctrine of informed consent/authorization was positioned at the center of reforms to post-mortem practice, it could reasonably be claimed to form the linchpin of the steps taken ostensibly to restore trust. Introducing the Royal Liverpool Children's Inquiry Report (2001) in the House of Commons, the then-Secretary of Health, Alan Milburn, maintained that:

> "The national health service can no longer assume that the benefits of science, medicine or research are somehow self-evident, regardless of the wishes of patients or their families. *The relationship between patients and the service today has to be based on informed consent.* That will require changes in practice, policy and medical education. As I have made clear today, it will also require changes in the law." (HP Deb [2000–2001] Vol. 362 col. 178. My emphasis)

Bell's (2006) caveat aside (see note 3), this emphasis on informed consent as a central principle was further reinforced through the introduction of penalties—fines and up to three years' imprisonment—for breaches of the Human Tissue Act 2004; and similar penalties apply in the Human Tissue (Scotland) Act 2006. It was perhaps inevitable that informed consent was rapidly identified as fundamental to reforming past practice, as the notion of individual autonomy resonates in contemporary bioethics (O'Neill 2002). Debate surrounding the nature and efficacy of informed consent is considerable (Corrigan 2003; O'Neill 2002, 2003; Stirrat and Gill 2005), but it should be recognized that parents themselves were vocal in their calls for the obligation to obtain informed consent to be enshrined in law, with attendant criminal sanctions. Despite the extant law failing to protect their rights, and a loss of trust in the law (Richardson 2004), parents perceived legislative change as a key step forward.

Set within the context of the 'audit explosion,' a key feature of society since the 1980s (Power 1997), the emphasis placed on informed consent and accountability in relation to post-mortem practice is compatible with government moves to modernize the NHS through the mechanism of clinical governance. Janus-faced, this preoccupation with regulatory forms of surveillance, in seeking to restore trustworthiness, may paradoxically also increase distrust by serving to highlight a culture of low trust (Power 1997). Nevertheless, Power (1997, 123) suggests that 'The audit society is only superficially a "distrusting society." Indeed, auditing is a practice which must be trusted and which is also itself, of necessity, trusting.'

Although this implies that a 'leap of faith' must ultimately be made, Harrison and Smith (2004, 375) contend that modernization policy in health and social care is premised on *confidence* rather than trust. Whether trust and confidence are distinctively separate concepts is a moot point. For Luhmann (1988, 97), confidence relates to those aspects of life that are taken for granted, whereas trust 'presupposes a situation of risk' and requires an active engagement on the part of the trustor. Smith (2005) mirrors Luhmann (1988) to a large extent, but specifically relates confidence to abstract systems and trust to interpersonal relations, arguing that current policies are designed to foster confidence in systems rather than trust in moral agents. According to Smith (2005, 309), therefore, systems, including the 'law, regulation, procedures, codes of conduct and expert knowledge,' reduce uncertainty and vulnerability at the macrolevel and thus *replace* trust as a medium of social exchange. Trust, by contrast, comes to the fore in those situations characterized by uncertainty and vulnerability, particularly at the microlevel (Smith 2005). Within this framework, particular importance is placed on the moral and affective features of trust, as opposed to the cognitive and rational (Harrison and Smith 2004; Smith 2005). It is argued that modernization policy privileges the latter over the former, leading to a focus on the provision of services rather than on an ethic of care. Smith (2005) and Harrison and Smith (2004) claim that this has negative implications for health and social care, highlighting in particular the potential hollowness of relationships based on an adherence to externally imposed rules and norms rather than moral values.

What are the implications of positing such a distinction between trust and confidence for establishing the efficacy of informed consent as a measure to restore trust? First, it calls into question to what extent the placing of informed consent at the center of reforms to post-mortem practice was a measure believed to be concerned with the restoration of trust. Although in the documentary data there were frequent references to a loss of trust and the need to restore trust, it is also the case that the term 'confidence' was regularly utilized in the same way, either separately from or alongside trust. In the following quotations for example, the first, from the CMO's National Summit, uses the term 'confidence' rather than 'trust,' and the second from the IRGROP uses both:

" . . . I am struck, as I think every doctor will be, by the amount of erosion of *confidence* in the medical profession. Much of what we have heard today I think underlines that erosion of *confidence*. I think medicine needs to take heed, indeed is now taking heed of this, and we need make sure that we try to rebuild that *confidence*." (Chief Medical Officer 2001, 51, my emphasis)

"Public *confidence* has clearly been severely shaken by the events which have unfolded over recent times both in Scotland and in England. It is vital that *trust* is re-established in order that relatives can be *confident* that they, and their relatives are treated with the utmost sensitivity by hospitals and that legitimate medical research is able to continue." (IR-GROP 2001, 7, my emphasis)

However, it is unclear whether such usage derives from a belief that confidence was either different from or the same as trust, that confidence would lead to trust, or is merely an artefact of language. As such, it cannot be readily ascertained whether it was felt that the proposed reforms would restore confidence or trust, or both. Harrison and Smith (2004, 375) are clear that in policy documentation 'the expectation of confidence is so embedded [. . .] that it almost defies exemplification.' The documentary data drawn on here however, encompasses a much wider range of material.

Second, and perhaps more fruitfully, they prompt deliberation of the potentially sterile relationships that might derive from privileging confidence over trust. An informed consent (or authorization) process that only fulfils a bureaucratic need for tick boxes, without promoting mutual communication and understanding, might meet the letter of the law, but certainly not the spirit of the law. Furthermore, to believe that doctors or other health care professionals were fulfilling their fiduciary duties only as a result of strict surveillance is a hollow reflection of the doctor–patient relationship, as it has been traditionally understood. As Möllering (2006, 63) argues, 'the idea of trusting or being trustworthy just because of external pressure is not seen as a durable basis for social interaction (except in rationalist accounts).'

Nevertheless, Möllering (2005, 290) believes control to be an integral part of trust, asserting that control assumes the existence of trust and trust assumes the existence of control. In relation to post-mortem practice it could be argued that greater control, in the form of legislation, regulation, and informed consent will provide structural assurance for parents and relatives that their wishes will be respected. In turn this will influence their positive expectations of individuals embedded within this overarching structure. As Möllering (2005, 290) contends, 'assuming the benevolence of another also assumes the particular social structures in which such benevolence is recognizable, relevant and thereby already shaped in a particular way. Hence trust also assumes the existence of control.' What is then crucial is how health care professionals use their remaining agency. If health care professionals use this to enhance communication with parents and relatives and demonstrate an empathetic understanding of their needs, then trust and control as a duality are integral to the reinstitutionalization of trust in post-mortem practice.

Thus far, I have analyzed the potential efficacy of the doctrine of informed consent in restoring trust by utilizing Möllering's (2001, 2005, 2006) perspective on trust and setting this against the existing literature, which relates specifically to health care. Particular attention has been paid to changes in the organizational culture of the NHS and their potential effects on trusting relationships at the macro- and microlevel. Overall, the steps taken to restore trust in the wake of the organ retention scandal can be perceived as moves to eradicate paternalism and to give greater autonomy to parents and relatives. However, as Corrigan (2003, 789) argues, 'The dualistic opposition between liberal concepts of freedom and autonomy versus powerful autocratic medical practices fails to recognise that power is not just a phenomenon that is exercised as an external constraint, but that prevailing cultural norms, values and systems of expertise shape the field of choice'. I suggest that these 'cultural norms, values and systems of exper-tise' are not only related to relationships of power but are also integral to relationships of trust. Therefore, I now highlight other discourses, beyond those of informed consent and autonomy, which were also evident in the documentary data, and potentially also influence trusting relationships in the context of post-mortem practice. These discourses, characterized by notions of the gift relationship and post-mortem citizenship, centered on the need for altruism to advance medical knowledge. Specifically, I consider whether attempts to link the concept of autonomy to notions of the 'gift relationship' and 'post-mortem citizenship,' which are inherently linked to our social responsibilities as members of a wider community, can, by grounding trust in an altruistic discourse, also facilitate a 'leap of faith.'

4.6   THE GIFT RELATIONSHIP AND POST-MORTEM CITIZENSHIP: GROUNDING TRUST IN ALTRUISM?

Post-mortem practice is substantively different from most other clinical situations in that it is not related to the treatment of individuals per se. Instead, it potentially offers a range of beneficial outcomes. These include: establishing the cause of death, giving certainty and perhaps comfort to relatives; providing medical information relevant to the existing or future health of family members (e.g., genetic diseases); furnishing knowledge of the efficacy of medical interventions, leading to improved care for future patients; and adding to a body of medico-scientific knowledge (Human Tissue Authority 2006; Laing and Becher 2006). In the case of fetuses and infants, a post-mortem may also provide information of relevance to future pregnancies (Laing and Becher 2006). The potential benefits are clear. However, those asked to give their informed consent, and indeed those who ask for it, cannot reliably know the nature and usefulness of the specific information that may be provided; there is always going to be an element of uncertainty. There are also longstanding concerns about the destruction of bodily integrity (Richardson 1987; Sanner 1994; Sheach Leith 2007). Thus, for at least some parents and relatives, the knowledge that a post-mortem and the subsequent retention of organs and tissues may bring has to be weighed against this loss (Richardson 2004).

As a result of the furore surrounding the organ retention scandal, considerable effort was made by a number of parties, including professional bodies and research institutions, to reinforce the benefits of post-mortem practice, not only to individuals but also to society as a whole. For example, in their submission to the Chief Medical Officer (CMO) in 2001, The Royal College of Pathologists argued that 'Pathologists performing post-mortem examinations were and are motivated to make reliable diagnoses to benefit families and future patients and *to improve the health of the nation by advancing medical knowledge*' (Royal College of Pathologists 2001, my emphasis). The rhetoric used by the medico-scientific community to promote the favourable outcomes of post-mortem practice bears great similarity to those made in respect of the public's participation in genetic research (Petersen 2005). In this context Petersen (2005, 284) argues that 'Words and phrases such as "altruistic," "gift," "sharing," "opportunities to help others," "common interest," "help those suffering from disease" and so on, have strong resonance in liberal democracies, especially with a broadening of the concept of social citizenship and an emphasis on citizen duties.' These terms also peppered the documentary data from the medico-scientific community in relation to post-mortem practice, providing a distinct counterbalance to the emphasis on autonomy and choice inherent in the discourse of informed consent. Therefore, although the decision to consent or not to consent to a hospital post-mortem and the subsequent retention of organs and tissues is an individual one, it is inherently linked to the wider social community and beliefs about citizenship. This also applies to judicial post-mortems where consent to retain material for purposes beyond establishing the cause of death is required. In this potentially altruistic framework, O'Neill (2002) problematizes the effectiveness of a narrow concern with informed consent alone for restoring trust, arguing that:

'Consent forms are not fundamental for restoring trust. Evidence that refusal is possible and respected, as well as tone, attitude and recognition of generosity are of greater importance. The generosity of those who give tissues, who allow research use of tissue that has to be removed and the generosity of relatives who give tissue *post mortem,* deserves gratitude. The best 'thank you' is not a legalistic form or an audit trail. If we merely construct more rigorous consent forms without showing gratitude where it is due we may improve trustworthiness, but we should expect no restoration of trust.' (O'Neill 2002, 160, emphasis in the original)

What would appear to be crucial for O'Neill (2002) is the basis of the trust relationship between those who ask for, and those who give their consent. Potentially, this is not a relationship solely based on the legalistic and surveillance aspects of informed consent but one also based in the acknowledgement of an altruistic act, and we can see here some similarities with Harrison and Smith's (2004) focus on the moral motivations of health care professionals. Reflecting Durkheim's philosophy on the basis of social order, O'Neill goes on to propose that 'If we seek to restore and maintain a culture of solidarity, and a better level of trust in the practices of removing, storing and using tissues, then we must aim for a *gift relationship* rather than for an audit trail' (2002, 158, emphasis in the original). Notions of the gift relationship are clearly articulated in one of the Chief Medical Officer's underlying principles for reforms to post-mortem practice:

'A gift relationship, the emphasis in all present legislation and guidance is on 'taking' and 'retaining.' The balance should be shifted to 'donation,' so that tissue or organs are given as a gift to help others and recognised as deserving of gratitude to those making donations.' (Department of Health, Department of Education and Employment, Home Office 2001, 37)

Shifting the emphasis, from consent to the *taking* of organs and tissues, to one of positive *donation* would, it is argued, 'signal a new relationship with the public and bereaved families' (Department of Health, Department for Education and Employment 2001, 41). Lock (2002, 318) argues that the gift metaphor has the effect of representing the act as a personal choice which, like the discourse of informed consent, privileges autonomy. Paradoxically, however, the gift relationship as constructed by Titmuss (1970) in his classic study of the motivations of blood donors also involves a social bond. This social bond and the existence of a wellspring of altruism was repeatedly invoked in the context of post-mortem practice. There was also a further related thread in the documentary data that focused on the requirement to consider our social responsibility to fellow citizens and the advancement of medical science in relation to our own deaths and/or of those close to us and to subscribe in effect to what I have coined a 'post-mortem citizenship.' The notion of post-mortem citizenship was articulated in discussions surrounding the correct 'balance' between the rights of the deceased, the rights of relatives and the needs of society as a whole, as in the Department of Health's Human Bodies, Human Choices (HBHC) consultation document:

'This report stresses the need to strike an acceptable balance between the rights and expectations of individuals and families and broader considerations, such as the importance of research, education, training, pathology and public health surveillance to the population as a whole.' (HBHC 2002, 1)

However, the consultation document itself was criticized by some for privileging the rights of the individual over the needs of society as a whole:

'We need to remember that "the good of all" is not an abstract concept but is actually composed of the rights and wishes of large numbers of individuals, whose needs must not be ignored. If we are to consider the balance between individuals and the public interest we must remember that in some circumstances, unthinkingly to respect the autonomy of a single individual may harm the autonomy of many.' (Response 42, HBHC 2002)

Outwith the documentary data, in the context of a discussion focusing on the extent to which consent is central to our ethical judgements, the notion of post-mortem citizenship is clearly articulated here by Evans:

' . . . there is, I think, an ideal of collective solidarity underlying the collective provision of health care free at the point of use [. . .] Enjoying the benefits of free health care brings responsibilities, and perhaps these extend beyond simply contributing through your national insurance payments. We do not (any longer) coerce people into taking part in medical research. And yet those who refuse to be research subjects while still enjoying the benefits of the best currently available treatments are, in effect, standing on the shoulders of research subjects in the past, but refusing to hold up the feet of patients in the future.' (2001, 825)

Again encapsulating the concept of post-mortem citizenship, similar sentiments were also expressed in the *Journal of Medical Ethics* (June 2003). Here, van Diest, Lopes Cardoso and Neising (2003, 135) state that in relation to tissue donation, 'the principle of solidarity should take priority over the right of self-determination here.' In addition, the pathologist Emson (2003, 3) argues that the body should become the responsibility of the state, and Harris (2003, 131) believes that 'The public interest in saving the lives of fellow citizens at risk is at least as urgent and as important as the public interest which justifies court ordered post-mortem examinations.' These arguments may be viewed as being at the furthest end of the continuum of attitudes towards the use of the deceased body, and as such, are unlikely to find favour in the contemporary climate.

Overall, notions of the gift relationship and post-mortem citizenship, although not diametrically opposed to the doctrine of informed consent, serve to highlight the context in which the act of giving consent takes place. I have argued elsewhere (Sheach Leith 2007) that these altruistic discourses may be invoked to promote the giving of consent for a post-mortem, and/ or the retention of organs and tissues, as a normative choice, but what is of importance here is to recognize their influence in shaping the discursive field within which a trusting relationship takes place. Brownlie and Howson (2005, 235) emphasize trusting in the context of mumps, measles and rubella vaccination as a 'complex relational practice that operates at a number of levels including the individual, interpersonal, institutional and socio-political.' As I have sought to demonstrate here, it is only by conceptualising trust in this way that can we begin to fully understand what might lead parents and relatives, through an active process of reason, routine and reflexivity, to suspend irreducible uncertainty and vulnerability and make a 'leap of faith.' The enshrinement of informed consent in legislative change, and the surveillance mechanisms now regulating post-mortem practice in the NHS, could strengthen the bases for trust, yet altruistic beliefs in the benefits accruing to humankind as a whole may also serve to reduce the existing cavernous chasm between the bases of trust and trust itself.

4.7   CONCLUSION

Trust once lost is not easily recaptured. Based on a potent mix of images of innocent child bodies, the perceived sanctity of the parent–child relationship, concerns about the potential of medical science to commodify the body, and haunted by the spectre of paternalism, the organ retention scandal brought relationships of trust to the fore. The doctrine of informed consent, placed at the center of reforms to post-mortem practice, carried the main burden for arguably restoring trust. However, the tighter regulation of professional practice has been revealed to be a double-edged sword. On the one hand, there is a concern that the macroprocesses of clinical governance only serve to change the basis of relationships in health and social care, from one of trust to one of confidence, with potentially negative effects (Harrison and Smith 2004; Smith 2005). In addition, the processes of audit and accountability, and surveillance and control, are themselves seen to be symptomatic of low levels of trust (O'Neill 2002; Power 1997). On the other hand, in the context of post-mortem practice, it could be argued that the same processes will provide greater structural assurance for parents and relatives that their wishes will be respected. In turn, this may strengthen the bases of trust—reason, routine and reflexivity—ultimately facilitating the reinstitutionalization of trust in post-mortem practice. Nevertheless, the notions of the gift relationship and post-mortem citizenship highlight the inherent tensions in seeking to restore trust through a concentrated focus on autonomy and informed consent by drawing attention to the significance of wider sociopolitical discourses. Grounded in altruism, the existence of these notions in the discursive field also influences the potential for trust in the context of post-mortem practice. Ultimately, taking all of the above into account, I would argue that the doctrine of informed consent *alone* is not enough to restore trust in post-mortem practice. Although it may support the bases of trust, by itself it cannot be the sole springboard for 'a leap of faith' or an 'act of suspension' (Möllering 2001, 2006).

This chapter has highlighted some of the challenges involved in understanding the nature of trust and its potential restoration in the wake of the organ retention scandal. The complexities of the trusting relationships involved, from trust in individuals to trust in institutions and ultimately to trust in the moral basis of the social order, make trust both vital and precarious. As post-mortem practice moves beyond its current troubled backdrop, further research is required to capture the active processes of routine, reason and reflexivity and the essence of the 'leap of faith' or 'act of suspension' that parents and relatives are asked to make when faced with this difficult choice. Continued exploration of the relationship between trust and control potentially also provides a fruitful avenue for enhancing existing conceptualizations of trust at the macro- and microlevels. Other potential research areas include the effects of the organ retention scandal on health care professionals. To what extent has this erosion of trust affected *their* trust relationships and what are the possible implications? Further empirical research is needed before we can fully comprehend the 'leap of faith' or 'act of suspension' that, in the context of post-mortem practice, is characterized in the opening quotation as an 'amazing gesture of trust and courage.'

NOTES

1. The documentary data included but was not limited to, Inquiry Reports; oral and written evidence submitted to the Inquiries; proceedings and publications of the Chief Medical Officer's National Summit and the Retained Organs Commission; as well as publications by professional bodies such as the Royal College of Pathologists, guidelines produced by the Department of Health and a large number of the responses to the Human Bodies Human Choices Consultation (2002). Illustrative of a move towards 'openness and transparency,' bar the latter, all the documentary evidence was publicly available. However, respondents to the HBHC (2002) consultation had given agreement for their responses to be made public and access to these was gained through the Department of Health.
2. These were The Royal Liverpool Children's Inquiry (1999); The Independent Review Group on Retention of Organs at Post-Mortem (Scotland; 2000); The Human Organs Inquiry (HOI) (Northern Ireland; 2001) and The Isaacs Inquiry (2001).
3. Bell (2006) argues that, as it is now permissible to perfuse the organs of nonheartbeating potential organ donors until the wishes of relatives can be ascertained, in this case, the principle of informed consent is surrendered.
4. Where a coroner's or procurator fiscal's post-mortem was conducted, with no prior contact with health care staff—for example, a case of sudden infant

88 *Valerie M. Sheach Leith*

death syndrome—further research is required to determine the nature of trust in this context.
5. See *AB and Others v. Leeds Teaching Hospital NHS Trust and Another* [2004] EWHC 644 (2004) QB.

REFERENCES

AB and Others v. Leeds Teaching Hospital NHS Trust and Another [2004] EWHC 644: (2004) QB.
Bell, M. D. D. 2006. The U.K. Human Tissue Act and consent: Surrendering a fundamental principle to transplantation needs? *Journal of Medical Ethics* 32 (5): 283–286.
Bennet, J. R. 2001. The organ retention furore: The need for consent. *Clinical Medicine Journal of the Royal College of Physicians* 1 (3): 167–171.
Bristol Royal Infirmary Inquiry. 2000. *The Inquiry into the Management of Care of Children Receiving Complex Heart Surgery at the Bristol Royal Infirmary: Interim Report Removal and Retention of Human Material.*
Brownlie, J., and A. Howson. 2005. 'Leaps of faith' and MMR: An empirical study of trust. *Sociology* 39 (2): 221–239.
Burkitt, I. 1999. *Bodies of Thought: Embodiment, Identity and Modernity.* London: Sage.
Calnan, M., and R. Rowe. 2005. Trust relations in the 'new' NHS: Theoretical and methodological challenges. 'Taking Stock of Trust,' ESRC Conference, London School of Economics, December 2005 [online], [cited 14 April 2007]. Available from <http://www.kent.ac.uk/scarr/events/Calnanand%20Rowe%20paper.pdf>
Campbell, A. V., and M. Willis. 2005. They stole my baby's soul: Narratives of embodiment and loss. *Medical Humanities* 31 (2): 101–104.
Chief Medical Officer. 2001. *National Summit Meeting on Organ Retention.* (11th January 2001).
Christensen, H. P. 2000. Childhood and the cultural construction of vulnerable bodies. In *The Body, Childhood and Society,* ed. A. Prout. Basingstoke: Macmillan.
Corrigan, P. O. 2003. Empty ethics: The problem with informed consent. *Sociology of Health and Illness* 25 (7): 768–792.
Department of Health, United Kingdom. 2002. *Human Bodies, Human Choices: The Law on Human Organs and Tissue in England and Wales. A Consultation Report.* London: Department of Health.
Department of Health, Department for Education and Employment, Home Office, United Kingdom. 2001. *The Removal, Retention and use of Human Organs and Tissue From Post-Mortem Examination. Advice from the Chief Medical Officer.* London: The Stationery Office.
Emson, H. E. 2003. Is it immoral to require consent for cadaver organ donation? *Journal of Medical Ethics* 29 (3): 125–127.
Erikson, E. H. 1963. *Childhood and Society.* New York: W. W. Norton and Co.
Evans, H. M. 2001. What's wrong with "retained organs"? Some personal reflections in the afterglow of "Alder Hey." *Journal of Clinical Pathology* 54 (11): 824–826.
Giddens, A. 1991. *The Consequences of Modernity.* Cambridge Polity Press.
Gilson, L. 2003. Trust and the development of health care as a social institution. *Social Science & Medicine* 56 (7): 1453–1468.
Hallam, E., J. Hockey, and G. Howarth. 1999. *Beyond the Body: Death and Social Identity.* London: Routledge.

Hansard Parliamentary Debates, United Kingdom, 5th ser., vol. 362, col. 178. 30th January 2001.

Harris, J. 2003. Organ Procurement: Dead Interests, Living Needs. *Journal of Medical Ethics* 29 (3): 130–134.

Harrison, S., and C. Smith. 2004. Trust and moral motivation: Redundant resources in health and social care? *Policy & Politics* 32 (3): 371–386.

Higonnet, A. 1998. *Pictures of Innocence, The History and Crisis of Ideal Childhood.* London: Thames and Hudson.

Human Organs Inquiry Report. 2002. United Kingdom. [online] [cited 4th June 2007) Available from <http://www.dhsspsni.gov.uk/index/hss/hoi-home/hoi-report.htm>

Human Tissue Act 1961 (c.54). London: The Stationery Office.

Human Tissue Act 2004 (c.30). London: The Stationery Office.

Human Tissue (Scotland) Act 2006: 2006 asp 4. London: The Stationery Office.

Illingworth, P. 2002. Trust: The scarcest of medical resources. *Journal of Medicine and Philosophy* 27 (1): 31–46.

Independent Review Group on the Retention of Organs at Post-Mortem. 2001. *Report of the Independent Review Group on the Retention of Organs at Post-mortem (Final Report From Phase One).* Edinburgh: The Scottish Executive.

Isaacs Report. 2003. *The Investigation of events that followed the death of Cyril Mark Isaacs.* London: The Stationery Office.

Laing, I. A., and J.-C. Becher. 2006. International perspectives: The role of the neonatal necropsy today: A Scottish perspective. *Neoreviews* 7 (4): 177–182.

Lock, M. 2002. *Twice Dead: Organ Transplants and the Reinvention of Death.* Berkeley: University of California Press.

Luhmann, N. 1988. Familiarity, confidence, trust: Problems and alternatives. In *Trust: Making and Breaking Cooperative Relations,* ed. D. Gambetta. Oxford: Basil Blackwell.

Lupton, D. 1996. Your life in their hands: Trust in the medical encounter. In *Health and the Sociology of Emotions,* eds. V. James and J. Gabe. Oxford: Blackwell.

Maclean, M. 2002. Letting go . . . Parents, professionals and the law in the retention of human material after post-mortem. In *Body Lore and Laws,* eds. A. Bainham, S. Day Sclater, and M. Richards. Oxford: Hart Publishing.

Möllering, G. 2001. The nature of trust: From George Simmel to a theory of expectation. Interpretation and suspension. *Sociology* 35 (2): 403–420.

———. 2005. The trust/control duality: An integrative perspective on positive expectations of others. *International Sociology* 20 (3): 283–305.

———. 2006. *Trust: Reason, Routine, Reflexivity.* Amsterdam: Elsevier.

O'Neill, O. 2002. *Autonomy and Trust in Bioethics.* Cambridge: Cambridge University Press.

———. 2003. Some limits of informed consent. *Journal of Medical Ethics* 29 (1): 4–7.

Petersen, A. 2005. Securing our genetic health: Engendering trust in UK Biobank. *Sociology of Health and Illness* 27 (2): 271–292.

Power, M. 1997. *The Audit Society: Rituals of Verification.* Oxford: Oxford University Press.

Prior, L. 1997. Following in Foucault's footsteps: Text and context in qualitative research. In *Qualitative Research: Theory, Method and Practice,* ed. D. Silverman. London: Sage.

———. 2003. *Using Documents in Social Research.* London: Sage.

Richardson, R. 1987. *Death, Dissection and the Destitute.* London: Routledge and Kegan Paul.

————. 2004. Narratives of compound loss parents' stories from the organ retention scandal. In *Narrative Research in Health and Illness,* eds. B. Hurwitz, T. Greenhalgh, and V. Skultans. London: Blackwell BMJ Books.

Richardson, E. H., and B. S. Turner. 2002. Bodies as property: From slavery to DNA maps. In *Body Lore and Laws,* eds. A. Bainham, S. Day Sclater, and M. Richards. Oxford: Hart Publishing.

Rowe, R., and M. Calnan. 2006. Trust relations in health care—the new agenda. *European Journal of Public Health* 16 (1): 4–6.

Royal College of Pathologists, Submission (101), Chief Medical Officer. 2001. *National Summit Meeting on Organ Retention* (11th January 2001)

Royal Liverpool Children's Inquiry. 2001. *The Royal Liverpool Children's Inquiry Report.* London: The Stationery Office.

Salter, B. 2004. *The New Politics of Medicine.* Basingstoke: Palgrave MacMillan.

Sanner, M. A. 1994. A comparison of public attitudes toward autopsy, organ donation and anatomic dissection: A Swedish survey. *Journal of American Medical Association* 271 (4): 284–288.

Scheper-Hughes, N., and L. Wacquant, eds. 2002. *Commodifying Bodies.* London: Sage.

Schoeman, F. 1980. Rights of parents, and the moral basis of the family. *Ethics* 91 (1): 6–19.

Sheach Leith, V. M. 2004. *Body Wholeness and the Infant: A Sociological Study of the Practice of Pathology.* Thesis (Ph.D.): The University of Aberdeen.

————. (2007). Consent and nothing but consent? The organ retention scandal. *Sociology of Health and Illness* 29 (7): 1023–1042.

Smith, C. 2005. Understanding trust and confidence: Two paradigms and their significance for health and social care. *Journal of Applied Philosophy* 22 (3): 299–316.

Stevens v. Yorkhill NHS Trust and Another [2006] ScotCs CSOH_143 (13 September 2006).

Stirrat, G. M., and R. Gill. 2005. Autonomy in medical ethics after O'Neill. *Journal of Medical Ethics* 31 (3): 127–130.

The General Medical Council (Submission 102), Chief Medical Officer (2001) *National Summit Meeting on Organ Retention* (11th January 2001).

The Human Tissue Authority. 2006. *Code of Practice—Post-mortem Examination, Code 3* [online], [cited 30 November 2006]. Available from <http://www.hta.gov.uk/guidance/codes_of_practice.cfm>

Titmuss, R. M. 1970. *The Gift Relationship: From Human Blood to Social Policy.* London: George Allen and Unwin.

Turner, B. S. 1996. *The Body and Society: Explorations in Social Theory.* Second Edition. London: Sage.

van Diest, P. J., N. W. J. Lopes Cardoso, and J. Neising. 2003. Cadaveric tissue donation: A pathologist's perspective. *Journal of Medical Ethics* 29 (3): 135–136.

5 The Nature of Reciprocity and the Spirit of the Gift
Balancing Trust and Governance in Long-Term Illness

*Alexandra Greene, Peter McKiernan
and Stephen Greene*

5.1 INTRODUCTION

Since the early 1980s, developments in health service policy and practice have prompted careful reevaluation of the nature and importance of trust relationships in health care contexts (Mechanic 1998). The issue of trust arises across a range of health care conditions and settings including acute and long-term health care provision and primary, secondary and community contexts. This chapter focuses on trust in relation to the secondary care provision for young people with diabetes. Recognition of rising mortality and morbidity associated with poor management of diabetes and a greater emphasis on high-quality services for children and young people (*The National Service Framework* 2005), raise a number of specific issues in relation to trust. This chapter is a collaborative piece of work that pulls together three disciplinary backgrounds—anthropology, management and medicine—to inform findings from an action research project, funded by the patient representative group, Diabetes UK. Carried out between 2002 and 2004, the aim of this project was to examine the experiences of interactions between young people with Type 1 diabetes (T1D) and health professionals in seven outpatient clinics in Scotland. The policy background to this research includes the drive to improve public trust in the National Health Service (NHS) by imposing tighter regulations on high quality diabetes care, synonymous with patient-centered diabetes care and the more general concern to improve trust at a personal level between individual patients and health professionals. Such relationships must be carefully navigated with adult diabetic patients, and additional complexities appear to arise with young people who have diabetes. In particular, we argue that a powerful discourse in the United Kingdom—and indeed in the West generally—that portrays teenagers as a deviant and risk-taking group, who in this case cannot be trusted to manage their diabetes successfully, appears to clash with the ethos in the NHS of greater trust between health professionals and patients.

Our analysis also draws on a study undertaken ten years earlier with many of the same health professionals, but a different cohort of young people.[1] Drawing on these earlier interviews allows us to highlight apparent changes in professionals' accounts (Greene 2000, 2001; Greene and Greene 2005) and to explore how these professionals understood such changes. The combination of different periods of time in social enquiry generates a micro-dynamic picture that captures the immediacy and complexity of real lives and the varied context through which they unfold. In particular, it allows us to explore how better understandings of trust between young people and health professionals might be developed to support young people's optimal self-management of diabetes and corresponding long-term health.

This chapter sets up the background of the growth of clinical governance in the diabetes setting and with it the philosophy of patient-centered diabetes care (National Diabetes Framework 2002). Or, in other words, it presents the idea that the medical focus on improved outcome measures in diabetes are underpinned by trust, often described as concordant partnership between patients and their health professionals. The chapter goes on to chart young people's and health professionals' accounts of their relationships with one another, where they meet three times a month in the hospital outpatient clinics. Their narratives help to illustrate their own situations, as young persons struggling to balance the events of their lives with having to manage a difficult illness, or as health professionals trying to balance the pressures placed on them to improve outcomes in young people, against their knowledge that adolescents are notoriously poor managers of their diabetes. We conclude by drawing on our interpretation of what these findings reveal about the nature of trust.

5.2   THE EMERGENCE OF CLINICAL GOVERNANCE AND THE FOCUS ON QUALITY HEALTH CARE

There has always been an awareness of clinical errors and malpractice in the United Kingdom, but systemic evidence about these has been collected only since the 1960s. Such errors were publicly debated in the 1990s with the high-profile inquiries of pediatric surgery at the Bristol Infirmary (Kennedy et al. 2001); organ retention at Alder Hey Hospital (Royal Liverpool Children's Inquiry 2001); and the case of the U.K. based GP, Harold Shipman (Lord Laming et al. 2005). These inquiries foregrounded concerns about trust in health professionals (Mechanic 2001; Segall 2000; Welsh and Pringle 2001), and with the publication of the Institute of Medicine's report, *To Err is Human* (Kohn et al. 2002), wide-scale policy and legal changes were initiated, culminating in the establishment of rigorous systems to regulate medical performance and reshape health professionals' conditions of work. Reforms to clinical practice came under the auspices of clinical governance and involved a reshaping of budgetary responsibilities and the development of general management and service frameworks (Scottish Executive Health Department 2000). The Commission for Health Improvement was developed to deal with clinical misconduct and to provide clear programs of quality improvement activities; it was regulated through clinical audit (NHS Executive, 1998). With the move towards the prevention of costly variation in clinical practice and outcomes, quality performance was assessed through data systems that collected performance related information (Davies and Mannion 1999). Underpinning these initiatives was the desire to destabilize medical autonomy, sometimes described as the 'club culture' (Klein 1998, 51) and thus, to open up the arena to public scrutiny:

> 'The culture of the future must be a culture of safety and of quality; a culture of openness and of accountability; a culture of public service; a culture in which collaborative teamwork is prized; and a culture of flexibility in which innovation can flourish in response to patients' needs.' (General Medical Council 2001, 51).

Yet, despite the embedding of this powerful rhetoric within the culture of the NHS, what appeared to be missing was the information on *how* to implement these policy changes. As Entwistle (2006) observes, there are complex forms of care in complex health care systems, which means the particularities of quality improvement can be equally complex and difficult to perform. Moreover, the full implication of quality improvement is still unclear given the growth of long-term illnesses since the 1950s and the current limit on resources (Ferlie and Shortel 2001). At the heart of the emerging critique of the 'scientific' measurements of clinical standards and the efficiency of audit (Salter 2005) was the sense that such developments revealed little about the nature and value of health systems, personal relationships and the behaviour of individuals. This reinforces Gilson's (2003) point that 'health systems are inherently relational and so many of the most critical challenges for health systems are relationship and behavioural problems.' (2003, 1453).

For some working in the NHS, quality care was already happening, and these measures, therefore, were merely part of the public bureaucracy to make the system seem more transparent (Black 1998). Nevertheless, such bureaucracy has social consequences; locking up time, personnel and resources. By themselves audit practices can seem mundane and an inevitable part of a bureaucratic process, yet, set against the larger picture they can take on the contours of a distinct cultural artifact (Strathern 2000). In other words, in the diabetes field, these practices often culminated in feelings of 'war-weariness' about a system that was constantly changing, where few felt they had any control and where it was felt that only the most entrepreneurial or resourceful could succeed (Greene 2000, 2001; Greene and Greene 2005).

Added to the artillery of clinical governance is the emphasis on patient-centered care; which is argued to be synonymous with high-quality health care. 'Good Medical Practice' (General Medical Council 2001), therefore, endorses greater openness with patients and the replacement of traditional and paternalistic styles of practice with greater consumer knowledge and shared responsibility for improved health and illness outcomes. Embedded in these expectations, however, is a precarious balancing act between health professionals who are relied upon to regulate and check illness outcomes and those patients who are trusted to manage their illness at home and away from the medical domain (Baier 1992; Davies and Mannion 1999). Perhaps understandably, the government's effort to reflect public concern and move towards clinical reform has sparked a tug of war between the state and the medical profession for control of the agenda setting. Both aim to address the protection of the consumer and the decline in the public's trust in doctors, but each constructs its policy from a rather different set of institutional structures and values (Salter 2005). What is at stake for the medical profession is not just the means for ensuring quality performance but the possibility to preserve some professional autonomy and the energy needed to deliver it.

5.3   YOUNG PEOPLE WITH DIABETES

The clinical governance measures described above prompted a flurry of diabetes-specific policies, such as the Scottish National Diabetes Framework (2002); The clinical standards for diabetes NHS and Quality Improvement Scotland (NHS QIS 2004). Yet, despite these developments, medical evidence continues to suggest the management of diabetes is poorest among adolescents (Morris et al. 1997). Adolescence is understood as a critical time for diabetics, as it is often associated with deterioration in glycaemic control (high blood sugar) which brings with it the potential for disease complications. Adolescence in general, however, has long been understood within biomedical discourse as a time of physiological changes, as well as of emotional and behavioral problems. This builds on the 'storm and stress' conceptualization of adolescence by the psychologist Hall (1904) in the early twentieth century, as well as Erikson's (1950) 'identity crisis'. Even today adolescence continues to be characterized as a phase of sexual frustration, social restrictions, conflict between the generations, and general risk-taking behaviour. Such notions led the sociologists Hill and Fortenberry (1992) to argue that adolescence has been constructed as a 'culture-bound syndrome,' or, in other words, as a constellation of symptoms that has been categorized as a disease and which cannot be understood apart from a specific culture (Rittenbaugh 1982).

In contrast to biomedical assumptions that puberty is a universal experience, sociocultural research has highlighted the multiple beliefs and attitudes associated with this life stage across different parts of the world. For example, a number of societies choose to mark the transition from childhood to adulthood as a celebration and a public event involving formalized rites of passage, but in the United Kingdom, adolescence is more likely to be seen as a 'be-twixt and between' affair, where individuals must learn to work out, on a rather ad-hoc, trial and error basis, cultural beliefs about their own social positioning. Today, adolescence in Britain continues to be understood as a disturbing and difficult developmental phase beleaguered by problems of substance abuse, crime and sexually transmitted disease. As Hill and Fortenberry argue, adolescence

> ' . . . is seen as the inevitable "risk" factor for these widespread problems as if the origins of these problems were innate to adolescents rather than a product of complex interactions of individual biology, personality, cultural preference, political expediency and social dysfunction [. . .] by creating adolescence as a developmental period defined by its problems, "adolescent health" becomes an oxymoron [. . .] and "medicalized" into a condition that is inherently pathological'. (1992, 73)

It is against this background that health professionals' belief that they are looking after patients with two difficult-to-manage conditions—diabetes and adolescence—can be understood.

5.4   THE NATURE OF TRUST

From the discussion so far it is evident that health professionals are faced with a medical dilemma in the treatment of this age group. On the one hand, there is a redefining of the nature and parameters of the health care encounter, and a shift away from patient–professional interactions based on deference and compliance to encounters characterized in terms of 'patient centeredness' (May and Mead 1999), 'shared decision making' (Charles, Gafni and Whelan 1999) and 'concordance' (Bissell, May and Noyce 2004). For professionals this necessitates an acknowledgement of the place of patient values and lifestyle factors in health care decisions and in turn an acceptance of patient-led discussions that might run counter to professional judgement. This new orientation evokes a set of moral values designed to encourage public trust (Uslaner 2002), albeit with the accompanying risk of making individuals vulnerable to medical exploitation (Warren 2001). Insofar as this does actually shape young people's perceptions of health care, such developments echo theoretical orientations in the social sciences which seek to recast the young as active practitioners of their own lives (James and Prout 1997; Jenks 1996; Brannen et al. 1994, Brannen and O'Brien 1996). It is also a move away from futuristic, developmental paradigms that focus on how young people will turn out in adulthood, rather than valuing the immediacy of their experiences as young people.

Yet, on the other hand, health professionals, as noted, are faced with a powerful western ideology which constructs adolescents as far from competent, reliable or trustworthy. For adolescents with diabetes, these beliefs are apparently bolstered by medical evidence which, as noted earlier, show this age group to have the poorest record of controlling diabetes.

At the heart of this relationship between health professionals and young people with diabetes is a conceptualization of interpersonal trust as one person's expectations of another's good intentions and expertise. Trust, however, needs to be underpinned by a suspension of doubt for the very reason that the person who trusts is always left potentially vulnerable because they can be taken advantage of by the person in whom they have placed their trust. (Baier 1986; Möllering 2001; Calnan and Rowe 2004; Hall 2005; Brownlie and Howson 2005). Relationships of trust, then, cannot be assumed to relate to unshifting dependency but depend on the partners weighing up the benefits and costs of cooperating with one another, as well as the possibility of questioning the other's beliefs and actions (O'Neil, 2002a).

To further understand the trust relations between young people and their health professionals, we also draw on the concept of reciprocity: in particular, Mauss's (1993) work in *The Gift* and Sahlins's (1972) idea of 'generalized reciprocity.' For Mauss, the essence of a long-term relationship is the mutual understanding that those in receipt of a gift are indebted (politically liable to the donor) and obliged to make some return in the future. At the heart of Mauss's work is the significance of social solidarity and mutual understanding between people. To describe the nature of social exchange that also exists in Western societies, Sahlins (1972) describes three types of reciprocity: first, 'negative' reciprocity or that which exists in an asymmetrical relationship, where one side, rather like an enemy, intends to take advantage of the other person's good will; second, 'balanced reciprocity,' or short-term, symmetrical relationships that exist for a specific purpose, such as wishing to buy something and handing over money in the expectation that one will receive what one has bought; third, 'generalized reciprocity' and the notion of giving without expectation of immediate return. This describes transactions that occur between participants in highly trustful, long-term relationships, transactions that facilitate common goals and harness cooperation between people. The essence of this notion is that generalized trust in others is based on social solidarity and altruism (Offe 1999) and the expectation that people will act in the other's best (collective) interest, whatever the outcomes of the relationship (Hall 1999). Exemplars are the donation of blood or parental relationships with children. The act is altruistic, but there is also the trust that one may receive gifts in kind in the future, such as one's children doing well or receiving a donation of blood in an emergency.

In the following data we draw on these theoretical ideas about trust and reciprocity to explore the ways in which trust can be conceptualized in outpatient clinics for young people with T1D. First, however, we offer some details about the study methodology.

5.5 METHODOLOGY

This interdisciplinary study incorporated the approaches of social anthropology, management and medicine to explore the interactions between health professionals and young people (age 13–25 years) with T1D in seven clinics across three Scottish regions. By examining the macro- and microcultural issues that affect health care practices we sought to identify strategies that could be used to tackle both inequalities in health service provision and diabetes outcomes in young people.

After gaining approval from the three regional Research Ethics Committees, we recruited key health professionals working in the seven clinics. The regions were selected to represent the social demography of Scotland and, in order not to bias the study, the researchers (AG and PM) were not informed of the different centre outcomes, that is, young people's glycaemic control. A number of talks were given in the diabetes centres to inform health professionals about the project and to invite their participation. Key health professionals then approached the young people to request if the researchers could carry out tape-recorded interviews with them and observe them in consultations with health professionals. All nineteen of the health professionals (including paediatricians, physicians, nurse specialists, and dieticians) and sixty-five of the sixty-six young people who were approached agreed to be observed and interviewed.

We used purposive sampling methods (i.e. we intentionally sought to interview subjects with certain characteristics) to ensure a range of demographic variables and experiences.

5.5.1 Qualitative Methods and Analysis

Qualitative methods are particularly useful when the subject of research is relatively unexplored and the research question is loosely defined or open ended (Greenhalgh, Helman and Chowdhury 1998). This research involved a range of methods: semi-structured interviews, direct observation (of consultations and postclinic medical meetings) and analyses of personal documents (medical files). The observations took place first and were followed by separate interviews (semi-structured) with health professionals and young people at a time and place of their own choosing. Direct observations (of young people in consultations with a range of multidisciplinary health professionals) allowed the researchers to gain a close and intimate familiarity with the participants and thus to obtain more detailed and accurate information from their separate interviews. The strength of carrying out observations and interviews with participants over long periods of time is that researchers can discover discrepancies between what participants say in interviews, what they believe should happen (in the clinic consultations) and what actually does happen.

Data analysis was based on constant comparative method, and the health professionals' and young people's accounts were analyzed separately (Silverman 1993). Each transcript was repeatedly inspected before open codes were applied to describe each unit of meaning. Through comparison across transcripts, the open codes were developed into higher order thematic categories to provide a framework for coding the transcripts. AG continually checked and modified the framework categories to ensure an adequate fit with the data, and SG independently validated the assignment of the data to the categories. Case study analysis (Mitchell 1983) was used to generate the key features from the group of young people and the group of professionals.

The theory of reciprocity allowed us to critically examine (Geertz 1973) the place of diabetes in the lives of both the young people and the health professionals and to acknowledge its variable significance. Our aim was to elucidate the deeper meanings that inform the participants' conversations and behaviour and, thus, to allow their subjective experiences to inform the analysis and explanation (Rosaldo 1993). We are grateful to the generosity of the participants in the field; the following accounts rest on our interpretation of the data.

5.6   FINDINGS

As noted, ten years ago, one of the authors undertook research looking at the relationship between young people with T1D and health professionals (Greene 2000, 2001; Greene and Greene 2005). At that time, before the full impact of clinical governance, staff (many of whom remain in the same posts) spoke of the importance of befriending young people and of encouraging their attendance at appointments through the building of long-term reciprocal relationships with them. Poor outcomes in diabetes among this age group were expected, and thus, it was a time for staff to 'wait and see' and to hope that young people would eventually 'see the light' and manage their diabetes once they reached adulthood. Young people, in comparison, focused on the benefits of staffs' friendliness, which seemed constant, regardless of the effectiveness of their diabetes control. 'Friendliness' was cited as particularly important in a country where it was perceived that adults rarely listened. In fact, in return, young people strove to build and preserve the reputations of the staff by covering up their dissatisfaction with care. Nevertheless, they were particularly frustrated at being stereotyped as 'tricky' adolescents rather than negotiators juggling the difficulties of being young and having diabetes. Risk-taking (poor management) was not the essence of being young but was usually a case of weighing up the benefits of running their sugars high (poor control) and avoiding the costs or dangers such as having a 'hypo' (which brings with it the possibility of losing consciousness) when driving.

Findings from the most recent study suggest that the impact of clinical governance has changed the focus of these reciprocal interactions. We argue that the dynamics of the relationship between the young people and their health professionals can be framed through the themes of clinical governance and medicalization. In what follows, we first explore young people's accounts and then those of the health professionals before discussing what these findings reveal about the nature of trust.

5.6.1 Young People's Accounts: Governance and the Young Diabetic

In the current study, it was evident from observing the young people during consultations and listening to their interviews with AG that they were frustrated with health professionals' pre-occupation with diabetes outcome measures. These were based on blood tests, taken three times monthly at each clinic appointment, which show a patient's average blood sugar control (glycated haemoglobin) over three months since their last appointment. Perhaps understandably, this method was sometimes referred to by patients as a 'lie detecting device.' Young people spoke about their fear of waiting to see staff and hearing the 'bad news' about their diabetes. Staff, many young people believed, were unaware of their anxieties, particularly if they had been diagnosed with diabetes for a number of years. Compared with the previous study, young people described staff as being too concerned with medical notes (which showed the results of blood tests taken during the appointment); and adding data to their computers; and not concerned enough with listening to their stories. Blood measurements were far too abstract for most young people and revealed nothing of the 'ups and downs' of their daily lives. What they wanted was time to speak about the specifics of their situations and how this impacted on coping with diabetes.

> **Young person:** They're nice, but you have this feeling that they don't really see you, all they see is the number [blood glucose reading] in your notes. It doesn't matter what's been going on in your life, that's how you're judged, as a number.

Although the design of our study enabled young people to talk about matters that were significant to them, the extent to which they were preoccupied by issues other than diabetes became increasing apparent as fieldwork progressed. Many of the young people were facing a range of personal and familial challenges that existed prior or subsequent to having diabetes. These included issues around sexuality; schooling and higher education (particularly the stress associated with continual assessment and exams);

economic hardship and redundancy; parental divorce; peer friendships and relationships with adults.

> Respondent: They [staff] think it's [diabetes] the main thing going on in your life, but it's not, it's just a tiny part.

A number were sympathetic to the pressures health professionals were under to improve their management.

> Respondent: It's not their fault . . . they're under a lot of pressure, but it's the wrong way around, because they've got to focus on the end result, your [blood glucose] control, but for me I've got to start at the beginning and juggle everything in my life with diabetes.

Although the need to contextualize diabetes in a way that did not define it as a key life experience for young people or as something which determined their life chances was a significant theme of the Scottish Diabetes Framework (Morris et al. 2002), many young people experienced professionals as doing the opposite. Indeed all the young people who took part in the study talked about feeling more comfortable with staff that took a holistic approach to diabetes and who appreciated that diabetes was just one of the many variables affecting youth on a daily basis. They, therefore, felt attuned to staff that personally acknowledged them in the waiting room by remembering their name, who reassured them in the face of 'good' or 'bad' news and who warmed them up by asking them about themselves. They then were able to relate this information to strategies to help them manage their diabetes.

> Interviewer: What do you mean by warming you up?

> Respondent: [Laughs] It's a bit like sex, it's better if you get to know each other first . . . so it's better to do that in the clinic, so you don't go in [to the consultations] and they ask you about your diabetes control straight away.

The continuity of seeing the same member of staff at each appointment allowed them time to build on the stories about their diabetes and, as a result, to develop trust. Solidarity and reciprocity between young people and health professionals promoted a sense of claiming or owning health-care relationships as a two-way process. Where these arrangements can evolve over time and are based on sustained, attentive and supportive relationships they are perceived positively. However, where these features are missing, or inconsistently applied, such as being referred to different or inexperienced staff at clinics, the regime of management and clinic attendance becomes a trial for young people. Findings from this study suggest not only that that the task of sustaining diabetes management over many years is a particular challenge for young people but that disadvantaged relationships with staff may work to outweigh the efforts young people and their support networks make towards rigorous management of diabetes.

Young people also made clear their frustration when health professionals blamed their 'poor control' on being adolescent. For young people, poor control was complex and made all the more so by hormonal changes at puberty, which made management difficult, and by the pressure adults placed on them to 'stand on their own two feet' and manage diabetes alone. A number of young people, particularly young males, were more likely to keep quiet about the support they received from their families, especially their mothers, for fear they would be labeled a 'mummy's boy.'

> **Respondent:** There's a lot of pressure on you to do everything yourself, but I don't think that's normal. It's normal to want people to support you if you've got a problem, and that doesn't change just because you're a teenager.

Normative interpretations of adolescence as an age-based disorder drew attention away from the other significant challenges in their lives which were outlined earlier. Moreover, while many health professionals related their management behaviour to risk-taking, and part of being adolescent, young people, like the young people in the study ten years earlier, were more likely to see themselves as master negotiators, balancing the complexities of their diabetes with their everyday lives.

> **Respondent:** It's like they think you've got two illnesses to control: being diabetic and being a teenager.

> **Respondent:** It's not like being a teenager makes me do crazy things with my control, it's more about just growing up and having to handle not having a hypo [hypoglycaemia, or low blood glucose] and falling over in front of your friends.

5.6.2   Health Professionals' Accounts and Perceptions of 'Normal' Adolescence

In the current study, implicit in the health professionals' interviews were the changes that performance assessment brought to their relationships with young people and other colleagues. On the one hand, assessment was important to not only protect patients from poor quality health care but to protect themselves from litigation. On the other hand, the challenges of balancing these procedures with rising patient numbers and limited resources had shifted the focus away from the patient and onto the health care organization. These difficulties were even more pertinent with a group known to be, as one health professional suggested, 'especially challenging' to look after. As noted, evidence shows that young people, compared with other ages, demonstrate the poorest management of diabetes, hence the idea that more time and energy is required from staff to gain young people's trust and to encourage them to attend clinic appointments so that their diabetes could be checked and regulated. The majority of professionals in the study, however, understood adolescence to predispose these patients to take dangerous risks with their bodies (e.g., omitting insulin, running blood sugars high). Such behaviors start, as one health professional explained it, the 'time-bomb' of microvascular changes, which in turn could lead to serious complications and the deterioration of long-term health. Embedded within these beliefs was the idea that 'normal' adolescents were naturally deviant and that 'good controllers' were somehow abnormal by being too well controlled. As one senior member of staff described it:

> Respondent: You expect teenagers to have poor control, it's part of their make-up at that age. In fact, in my experience adolescents with good control are abnormal; I would say even a little bit worrying.

> Interviewer: How do you mean?

> Respondent: Well for example, they have a good relationship with their parents and get on with adults and want to do well. In my experience they can be a bit obsessive; overanxious. One young man used to bring a clipboard with all his results on including everything he'd eaten.

> Interviewer: You don't want them to do that?

> Respondent: We don't want to make them neurotic, no.

Implicit in these ideas is the understanding that the rigorous behaviour they might welcome in an adult patient would be considered deviant in an adolescent patient. Moreover, poor control, despite its long-term effects, was preferable to young people becoming over anxious.

For staff, patient-centred relationships (involving good outcomes through good relationships with patients) were perceived as essential to override any rebelliousness and anti-adult authority behaviour and underpinned young people's attachment to staff and their desire to attend clinic appointments. The rationale here was that if their behaviour could not be changed, at least staff could keep an eye on any physiological damage that might occur with the hope of nipping any early signs of deterioration in the bud. Encouraging this patient group to attend, however, required, as noted, a particularly high level of energy.

> **Respondent:** I think you've got to be a certain type of person to want to work with teenagers. It can be a thankless, soulless task and it can feel as if you're banging your head against the wall. And it's not about knowledge, they all know an incredible amount about diabetes and what they're doing to themselves [. . .] you have to be incredibly patient because most of the time its a case of building a relationship with them to keep them on board until they're older and want to start looking after themselves.

> **Interviewer:** Why do you think that is?

> **Respondent:** I don't think anyone has the answers, but in my experience it seems to be something to do with ownership of their own lives and taking on responsibility, like having a partner, children and having a mortgage. Our responsibility is to keep them as well as possible until they have this shift in perspective.

Most professionals agreed that national policy on 'patient-centered care' was right, but most were also frustrated by the lack of advice on how to implement the policy and how to create such relationships with this age group. From a practitioner perspective, therefore, the policy focus on 'patient-centeredness,' appeared to have more to do with improved outcomes than how to work with patients to achieve them.

> **Respondent:** No one would disagree that we need to improve diabetes outcomes, but that doesn't just happen naturally. You've got to work hard at gaining their respect; it takes energy to build the chemistry you need between you to make it work. They've got to feel it's worth doing all the things we ask them to do (insulin injections, blood tests, diet, exercise). I doubt half of us could do what we ask of our patients, if I'm honest. It takes an incredible amount of trust to get them to do what you ask, day in and day out, for the rest of their lives.

In fact, for some professionals the emphasis on collecting data to demonstrate that targets were being met reduced the time needed to work with patients to achieve these targets. Regulation for some, therefore, had rendered the intimacies of their relationships with patients invisible and replaced these with a focus on complex audit systems and mounting paper trails.

> **Respondent:** It's a good thing [audit], definitely, but I think it's got a bit out of hand. There's so much paperwork now it makes it more difficult to focus on the patients.

Respondent: It's becoming all about ticking boxes not patient-centered [. . .] and um, sometimes it's overwhelming and I wonder where the human part, the patient–carer relationship has gone.

5.6.3 Health Professionals' Perceptions of Service Change and Trust

An unexpected finding relating to regulation (not evident in the earlier study) was the apparent breakdown of trust not only between the staff in the different centres but also between staff and the NHS as an organization.

Respondent: Sometimes you wonder what's the point [in changing] it will only change back again in a few years. I've been in it [the NHS] long enough to know these things are always cyclical.

In fact, most professionals believed that diabetes services were already an exemplar of good standards and a 'pathfinder' for other services, and as such, much of the paraphernalia associated with audit was unnecessary. The creation of league tables had challenged the openness between centres and so the opportunity to share information and swap stories was lost; for professionals, this openness appeared to have been replaced with feelings of mistrust and competition. For a small number, however, the positive side of audit far outweighed these negative issues, with governance linked to public responsibility and the morality of health provision. For these professionals, any discord could be overcome by the powerful ethos of good will, solidarity, altruism and trust in and between clinicians and the willingness of clinicians to make sacrifices to advance medicine for the good of the patient:

Respondent: I feel strongly that we need to think about diabetes more holistically[. . .]. To improve care we need to think about prevention and effect; its relation to CHD [coronary heart disease], obesity, kidney failure, blindness etc. Standards are essential to move that along.[. . .] How can we achieve that if we don't know what's going on in Scotland? It's about laying our cards on the table and knowing where we have to make the changes and improve things.

Respondent: I feel passionately that we're moving in the right direction. It's an uncomfortable move for a lot of people, I know that. I sit on the XX Standards Board and its difficult [. . .] we're not used to it [audit] as a profession. But to me it's worth it to advance diabetes care. That's got to be a good thing.

For the majority of staff, however, audit had set centers up against each other, and had altered the delicate system of support, camaraderie and trust between members in the different centers:

Respondent: You could always trust your neighbour [another clinic] and share difficulties and ask for advice, but that's changed now because everyone is looking over the other's shoulder.

Respondent: I entered medicine to help people. The league tables have changed that ethos. I'm having to be an expert accountant and manager too because everyone is competing and out for themselves.

Interviewer: Can you give me an example?

Respondent: Yes, in the last audit, X had the best outcomes in Scotland [outcomes in young people]. The reaction in one of the clinics was that X must be cheating, you know, collecting the wrong bloods to get better outcomes. Now, I don't for one moment believe that was the case, but the point is that you would never have seen that sort of reaction before [. . .] everyone would have been pleased and asking them for tips.

5.6.4   Health Professionals' Accounts of Autonomy

For many professionals, particularly doctors, governance was viewed as a top-down system that altered the balance of professional autonomy and independence:

Respondent: There's a paradox here, you can't take away professional autonomy with one hand and with the other give us all this responsibility to take decisions about other people's lives [. . .] There's a misfit. You can't fight your corner on behalf of the patient if you don't have some power and independence.

Respondent: We're all fighting for money, for our little patch of expertise so you're not going to buy into something if you don't think it's going to fit your needs. To give you an example, I'm interested in retinopathy services in the community, but my colleague in X is more involved in foot care. If you don't feel what you're being asked to do will give you something personal in return then you just end up paying lip service to the system.

However, another clinician, a nurse manager, described medical independence rather differently:

Respondent: Doctors see themselves as more independent than us [nurses] [. . .] and trying to organize them can feel like herding cats.

For a small number, getting involved on the regulatory committees was a move to reintroduce a sense of agency and ownership. Their involvement allowed them to feel they were moulding the system to the specifics of the diabetes services, rather than merely being on the receiving end of it. For these professionals, pragmatic collusion was realistic and a necessary political action, a case of 'If you can't beat them it's better to join them.'

Committee work was perceived as offering respectability, professional development, and the possibility of merit awards and, importantly, some time out from the pressurized 'coal-face.' Many spoke about feelings of professional 'burnout' and the tedium of looking after a long-term illness that was difficult to control. Time-out provided a change and variety in a job that was pressurized and, at times, monotonous and demoralizing: 'If I'm honest the [committee] work provides a fillip from the daily grind of the work.'

However, time off for some left others to cover the clinical load. Moreover, the products of these committees could be more regulations and paper trails for those at the coal-face:

> Respondent: Ok, we do need to be regulated, everyone would agree with that, but the more they work on these committees the more they send down to us, and we're the ones that have to try to cope with the mountains of paper work.

This was particularly relevant for nursing staff and other affiliated professions who had less opportunity to join medical committees, and this may, in part, account for the high levels of sick leave among them. Partaking in governance initiatives therefore appeared to be an opportunity for some and not for others. For the more sceptical, regulations enforced hierarchical relationships between managers and health professionals and reinforced structures of competition. Moreover, these regulations were often embedded within a no-can-do environment of fractured collegial relationships that many felt wore away at staff's energy levels and their drive to be creative and entrepreneurial. Of importance to these professionals was the overall effect they perceived these factors to be having on their relationships with young people. Many were worried that the focus on organizational issues, such as outcome measures, gave young people the impression that they were not interested in their lives.

For these professionals, reciprocity between professionals and young people was crucial to working with an illness where burnout—'diabetes fatigue'—was common and where limited resources, rising patient numbers and sub-optimal outcomes in adolescents contributed to the demoralization of both young people and health professionals. Reciprocity offered a way of containing these difficulties, when faced with this high-risk illness, as it facilitated disclosures by young person, and as a result encouraged the successful management of diabetes (Bandura 1993; Mechanic 1998).

5.7   DISCUSSION

Successful management of diabetes requires that service providers understand the lifestyle, beliefs and attitudes of the patients being treated (Greenhalgh et al. 1998). This chapter describes how the shift from self-regulatory approaches in medicine to a government-driven, interventionist style shaped the experiences of professionals and patients. Yet the importance of these experiences is rarely featured in the formalistic approaches to health care evaluation.

Though a small number of health professionals were willing to put their trust in the new system of governance, the majority gave accounts of how patient-centered ideology had become inextricably bound by policy to the rationalistic and bureaucratic discourse of regulation (Mackintosh 2000). Implicit in their narratives was a concern to achieve quality care in a way that allowed them to maintain their enthusiasm for working with this age group. What was frustrating for many of these professionals, however, was the obvious mismatch between assessing young people's physical health and their social and psychological well-being. The latter involved employing hunches, intuition and empathy—skills which are impossible to audit. Consequently, management systems ignored the time and energy needed for reflection and creativity to nurture reciprocal and trusting relationships with the young. Moreover, the drive for league tables fractured the delicate balance of trust between health care centers.

Supporting these findings, young people, too, spoke of their perceptions that health professionals were preoccupied with checking their diabetes measures. This implied that diabetes *was* the event that defined their young lives, rather than part of an ongoing social process that was played out in a complex variety of ways, over time. From the young people's perspectives, this preoccupation increased professionals' negative attitudes to young people and fed in to the construction of young diabetics as a homogeneous group of risk-takers who were unsuccessful managers of their illness. Pertinent here is the social positioning of adolescents, compared with adults, as influenced by inherent power relations embedded in medical practice (Young et al. 2003). The young people's accounts highlight the extent to which they are major actors in developing trust relations and how long-term trust and reciprocity cannot be driven by adult knowledge and priorities.

5.7.1   The Nature of Reciprocity and the Spirit of the Gift

Since the 1970s, patient initiatives in the United States and Europe have asserted the claim that patients need to be regarded as experts on their own illness. More recently, patients have been expected to take an active role in their own care and to be treated as equal stakeholders in the policy debate. Yet, even as evidence-based medicine advocates improving patient care, the methods used to define outcomes remain firmly in the hands of the experts (Tomes 1999).

Against the powerful discourse of clinical governance, it can be difficult to make a case for the role of trust and reciprocity in long-term illness. This is particularly so when target setting, key to surveying and measuring performance, is the basis of governing at a distance and appears to make the intimacies of relationships redundant (Flynn 2002).

Yet, trust is clearly an issue both for health professionals who trust young people to return to clinic and for young people who trust staff's continual need to check their blood. Systems of trust, as with those of governance, are socially situated and constructed within the particularities of relationships. Trust, however, compared with governance, is complex because of the very fact that it is symbolic and thus dynamic and, accordingly, in a constant state of transformation. It can never, therefore, be an assumed or dictated part of the health care system. Here, trust is practical and necessary to secure long-term relationships where risk is associated with uncertain youth behaviour and, as a result, uncertain disease outcomes. The creation of solidarity, good relations and mutual understanding between various clinic centers and between patients and health professionals are seen as key gifting relationships (Malinowski 1978). These are reciprocal relationships based on networking and exchanging information, support, gossip, and anxieties (Mauss 1993). Health professionals appear to work according to the principles of generalized reciprocity: support is given, regardless of the young person's diabetes outcome (Sahlins 1972). The young people, too, must appreciate that blood checking is necessary and reliable; they are in receipt of 'the gift' and hence are indebted (politically liable to the donor/health professional) and obliged to make a return (Mauss 1993). So far as the young people in this study are concerned, this manifests itself as a sense of commitment to the health carers. Social solidarity amongst young people and health professionals is key to delivering altruistic care. This is a form of care where everyone's contribution should be valued and respected and where trust is built on the basis of good faith rather than jural sanctions. Hierarchy, though not absent, is low-key so that everyone's role in the partnership can be maximized.

What makes this interaction reciprocal is the sense of satisfaction the giver feels and the social closeness that 'the gift' fosters (Mauss 1993). Between people who engage in generalized reciprocity, there is a maximum amount of trust and a minimum amount of social distance. Entwistle states that trust between people is generally strengthened in reciprocation and that patients are more likely to trust in health professionals who demonstrate trust in them (Entwistle 2006). More specifically, trust between health professionals and young people with diabetes offers a foundation for long-term dialogue and a chance to confront and work through any differences, with the hope of encouraging self-reflection and change.

This study, informed by the health practitioners' and young people's voices, suggests that there is a misfit between such notions of trust and reciprocity and the new audit culture. Indeed, governance, which by its very nature depends on measurements and monitoring, is put in place to override reliance on interpersonal trust. Yet attempting to renegotiate relationships between young people and health professionals can create mistrust and make it more likely that young people will not attend clinics so that measurements can be taken in the first place. The counterbalance does not mean the abandonment of regulation but the recognition that interpersonal trust should never be overridden by external drivers in the NHS. Although the time put into interdependent relationships may seem costly, we argue that our data indicates that the investment in such relationships is crucial to underpin the sustainability of a quality culture in the NHS.

NOTES

1. The study referred to here was carried out between 1996 and 2000 and formed part of AG's Ph.D. research (Greene 2000). The study was invited by the Hvidore Study group (Hvidore 1997) to examine the sociocultural differences between international diabetes centres with vastly different outcome measures in young people with diabetes. The use of data from the earlier study on the Scottish Diabetes Centre in this chapter is intended to provide some background to the changes we have identified in the relationships of trust between young people and health professionals over the last decade.

REFERENCES

Baier, A. C. 1986. Trust and antitrust. *Ethics* 96 (2): 231–260.
———. 1992. The Tanner Lectures on Human Values, *Trust,* Princeton University, Princeton, NJ, 68 March 1991 [online]. Available from: <http://www.tannerlectures.utah.edu/lectures/baier92.pdf>
Bandura, A. 1993. Perceived self-efficacy in cognitive development and functioning. *Educational Psychologist* 28 (2): 117–148.
Bissell, P., C. R. May, and P. R. Noyce. 2004. From compliance to concordance: Barriers to accomplishing a re-framed model of health care interactions. *Social Science Medicine* 58 (4): 851–862.
Black, N. 1998. Clinical governance: Fine words or action? *British Medical Journal* 326: 297–298.
Brannen, J., K. Dodd, A. Oakley, and P. Storey. 1994. *Young People, Health and Family Life.* Buckingham: Open University Press.
Brannen, J., and M. O'Brien. 1996. *Children and Families.* London: Falmer Press.
Brownlie, J., and A. Howson. 2005. Between the demands of trust and government: Health practitioners, trust and immunization work. *Social Science and Medicine* 62 (2): 433–443.
Calnan, M., and R. Rowe. 2004. Social capital in Britain. *British Journal of Political Science* 29 (3): 417–462.
Charles, C., A. Gafni, and T. Whelan. 1999. Decision-making in the physician–patient encounter: Revisiting the shared treatment decision-making model. *Social Science Medicine* 49 (5): 651–661.
Davies, H. T. O., and R. Mannion. 1999. Clinical governance: Striking the balance between checking and trusting. In *Reforming Markets in Health Care—An Economic Perspective,* ed. P. C. Smith, Open University Press. (Also reproduced

as Clinical governance: Discussion Paper 165. Centre for Health Economics, University of York: U.K.).

Entwistle, V. A., and O. Quick. 2006. Trust in the context of patient safety problems, *Journal of Health Organisation and Management* 20 (5): 397–416.

Erikson, E. 1950. *Childhood and Society*. New York: Norton.

Ferlie, E. B., and S. M. Shortell. 2001. Improving the quality of healthcare in the United Kingdom and United States: A framework for change. *The Milbank Quarterly* 79 (2): 281–315.

Flynn, R. 2002. Clinical governance and governmentality. *Health, Risk and Society* 4 (2): 155–173.

Geertz, C. 1973. *The Interpretation of Cultures. Thick Description: Towards an Interpretative Theory of Culture*. USA: Basic Books.

General Medical Council. 2001. *The Bristol Case: A serious departure from safe professional standards* [online], [cited April 2001]. Available from: <http://www.bristol-inquiry.org.uk>

General Medical Council, Protecting Patients Guiding Doctors. 2001. *Good Medical Practice*.

Gilson, L. 2003. Trust and the development of health care as a social institution. *Social Science and Medicine* 56 (7): 1453–1468.

Greene, A. 2000. Health carers' and young peoples' conceptualisations of chronic illness: An anthropological interpretation of Diabetes Mellitus. Unpublished Ph.D.: Department of Social Anthropology, University of Saint Andrews, Scotland.

———. 2001. Cross cultural differences in the management of children and adolescents with diabetes. *Hormone Research* 57 S1 (2): 75–77.

Greene, S., and A. Greene. 2005. Changing from the paediatric to the adult service: Guidance on the transition of care. *Journal of Practical Diabetes* 22 (2): 41–46.

Greenhalgh, T., C. Helman, and A. M. Chowdhury. 1998. Health beliefs and folk models of diabetes in British Bangladeshis: A qualitative study. *British Medical Journal* 316: 978–983.

Hall, G. S. 1904. *Adolescence: Its Psychology and its Relations to Psychology, Anthropology, Sociology, Sex, Crime, Religion and Education*. New York: Appleton.

Hall, M. A. 2005. The importance of trust for ethics, law and public policy. *Cambridge Quarterly of Healthcare Ethics* 14 (2): 156–167.

Hall, P. A. 1999. Social capital in Britain. *British Journal of Political Sciences* 29 (3): 417–462.

Hill, R. F., and J. D. Fortenberry. 1992. Adolescence as a Culture-Bound Syndrome. *Social Science and Medicine* 35 (1): 73–80.

James, A., and A. Prout. 1997. *Constructing and Reconstructing Childhood*. Basingstoke: Falmer Press.

Jenks, C. 1996. *Childhood*. London: Routledge.

Kennedy, I., B. Jarman, R. Howard, M. Maclean, et al. British Royal Infirmary Inquiry. 2001. *Learning from Bristol: The report of the public inquiry into children's heart surgery at the Bristol Royal Infirmary 1984–1995*. London: The Stationary Office.

Klein, R. 1998. Editor's choice: The dark side of medicine. *British Medical Journal* 316.

Kohn, L. T., J. M. Corrigan, and M. S. Donaldson. 2000. *To Err Is Human: Building a Safer Health System*. Committee on Quality of Health Care in America, Institute of Medicine.

Lord Laming of Tewin, Smith, J., et al. 2005. *The Shipman Inquiry*. Crown Copyright.

Mackintosh, M. 2000. Do health care systems contribute to inequalities? In *Poverty, Inequality and Health: An International Perspective*, eds. D. Leon and G. Walt. Oxford: Oxford University Press.

Malinowski, B. 1978. *Argonauts of the Western Pacific: an Account of Native Enterprise and Adventure in the Archipelagos of Melanesian New Guinea.* London: Routledge and Keegan Paul.

Mauss, M. 1993. *The Gift, the Form and Reason for Exchange in Archaic Societies.* London: Routledge.

May, C., and N. Mead. 1999. Patient-centeredness: A history. In *General Practice and Ethics: Uncertainty and Responsibility*, eds. C. Dowrick and L. Frith, 76–90. London: Routledge.

Mechanic, D. 1998. Public trust and initiatives for new health care partnerships. *Millbank Quarterly* 76 (2): 281–302.

———. 2001. The managed care and backlash: Perceptions and rhetoric in health care policy and the potential for health care reform. *The Milbank Quarterly* 79 (1): 35–54.

Mitchell, J. C. 1983. Case and situation analysis. *Sociological Review* 31 (2): 187–211.

Möllering, G. 2001. The nature of trust: From Georg Simmel to a theory of expectation, interpretation and suspension. *Sociology* 35 (2): 403–420.

Morris, A., et al. 2002. (Scottish Diabetes Group) Scottish Executive Health Department. *Scottish Diabetes Framework: The Blueprint for Diabetes Care in Scotland in the 21st Century* [online], [cited April 2005]. Available from: <http://www.diabetesinscotland.org/diabetes/maintainPages/DownloadablePub.asp>

Morris, A. M., D. I. R. Boyle, A. D. McMahon, S. A. Greene, T. M. MacDonald, and R. W. Newton. 1997. For the DARTS/MEMO Collaboration. Adherence to insulin treatment, glycaemic control and ketoacidosis in *IDDM Lancet* 350: 1505–1510.

Mortensen, H. B., and P. Hougaard. 1997. International perspectives in childhood and adolescent diabetes: A review. The Hvidøre Study Group on Childhood Diabetes. *Journal of Pediatric Endocrinology and Metabolism* 10 (3): 261–264.

NHS Executive. 1998–2005. Information for health: An information strategy for the modern NHS. A national strategy for local implementation, Department of Health, NHS Executive. 1 September 1998.

NHS Quality Improvement Scotland. 2004. *NHS QIS National Overview—Diabetes.* Edinburgh Office [online], [cited April 2005]. Available from: <www.nhshealthquality.org>

Offe, C. 1999. How can we trust our fellow citizens? In *Democracy and Trust*, ed. M. E. Warren. Cambridge: Cambridge University Press.

O'Neill, O. 2002a. *A Question of Trust: The BBC Reith Lectures 2002.* Cambridge: Cambridge University Press.

Redfern, M., J. Keeling, E. Powell, et al. 2001. *The Royal Liverpool Children's Inquiry Report.* The Honorable the House of Commons Committee.

Rittenbaugh, C. 1982. Obesity as a culture bound syndrome. *Culture, Medicine and Psychiatry* 6 (4): 347–361.

Rosaldo, R. 1993. *Culture and Truth. The Remaking of Social Analysis.* Boston: Beacon Press.

Royal Liverpool Childrens' Inquiry. 2001. The Royal Liverpool Children's Inquiry Report. London: The Stationery Office.

Sahlins, M. 1972. *Stone Age Economy.* New York: Aldine De Gruyter.

Salter, B. 2005. *Governing UK Medical Performance: A Struggle for Policy Dominance, from Governing Doctors: A Comparative Analysis of Pathways of Change*, working paper.

Scottish Executive Health Department. 2000. *Our National Health: A Plan for Action, A Plan for Change.* Edinburgh: The Stationery Office.

Segall, M. 2000. From cooperation to competition in national health systems—and back? Impact on professional ethics and quality of care. *International Journal of Health Planning and Management* 2000 15 (1): 61–79.

Silverman, B. 1993. *Interpreting Qualitative Data: Methods for Analyzing Talk, Text and Interaction.* London: Sage.

Strathern, M. 2000. *Audit Cultures: Anthropological Studies in Accountability, Ethics and Academy.* London: Routledge.

The National Service Framework for Children, Young People and Maternity Services. 2004. Standard 10; Section 8.

Tomes, N. 1999. From patients' rights to consumers' rights: Historical reflections on the evolution of a concept. Making history: Shaping the Future—Proceedings of the 8th Annual The MHS Conference 1998: Hobart.

Uslaner, E. 2002. *The Moral Foundation of Trust.* Cambridge: Cambridge University Press.

Warren, M. E. 2001. *Trust in democratic institutions.* Paper prepared for the European Research Conference (EURESCO) on Social Capital: Interdisciplinary Perspectives. UUK: Exeter: 15–20 September 2001.

Welsh, T., and M. Pringle. 2001. Editorial. Social capital: Trusts need to recreate trust. *British Medical Journal* 323: 177–178.

Young, B., M. Dixon-Woods, K. C. Windridge, et al. 2003. Managing communication with young people who have a potentially life threatening chronic illness: Qualitative study of patients and parents. *British Medical Journal* 326: 305.

6 Accountability and Trust in Integrated Teams for Care of Older People and People With Chronic Mental Health Problems

Guro Huby

6.1 INTRODUCTION: DILEMMAS OF TRUST AND ACCOUNTABILITY IN HEALTH CARE ORGANIZATIONS

6.1.1 Trust and the Health Services

Trust has emerged as a major issue in the organization and delivery of health services world-wide. In the United Kingdom, several incidents described elsewhere in this volume have sparked off high-profile public inquiries which have brought to the fore questions about the safety of health care and the level of public trust in health services.

The ferocity of these debates is noteworthy when set against the backdrop of a general reduction of life-threatening health hazards in developed economies such as that of the United Kingdom. Beck (1992) links the increased concerns with 'risk' and an accompanying erosion of trust to the advances in scientific knowledge and techniques and a rise in the reliance on experts. Moreover, a global economy has weakened the post-World War II consensus, which was based on the provision of community-sustaining services at a national level, and moved the responsibility for health, education, work and safety on to individuals who now make their own contracts with chosen experts and providers. The current preoccupation with trust, therefore, is clearly not only a matter of the number and magnitudes of breaches. It is also related to social change and the way hazards, and refuge from them, are framed and defined in new contexts and by new protagonists.

In the United Kingdom, one answer to these debates has been to put systems in place that require practitioners and organizations to account for their safe practice and competence (Dept. of Health 1998). This chapter will examine how systems of accountability rebound in various ways on the social construction of trust in health care. There is a growing interest in accountability and the construction and erosion of trust between providers and users of health care (e.g., Davies 1999), but less is known about how trust is constructed, maintained or undermined in relationships among staff, and how systems of accountability impact on these relationships. This chapter focuses on the latter and presents an example from the 'integrated' health care setting in Scotland. It also draws general implications for ways in which the relationship between accountability and trust among practitioners may be managed in health care settings undergoing change.

6.1.2   What is 'trust'?

The symbolic nature of 'trust' makes it difficult to capture. Rowe and Calnan (2006) argue that because 'trust' has been ignored theoretically, conceptual clarification has been neglected. 'Trust' has been confused with other related dimensions such as confidence (Checkland, Marshall and Harrison 2004), alienation, solidarity and participation. Luhmann (1979) saw 'trust' as socially produced and a means of reducing complexity. In order to make the world manageable, individuals have to agree on, and put trust in, one of a vast number of possible definitions of a social situation as the basis of action. Trust is thus fundamental to human organization. According to Garfinkel (1967) it goes to the heart of the moral order—to our reason to take for granted a wide range of features of the social order and, as a consequence, our place in it.

Garfinkel's view on 'trust' emerged from his theory of ethnomethodology or the methods whereby we construct our everyday worlds. Central to his theory is the way people account for themselves, their actions and motivations, and the way these accounts can be interpreted and understood. According to Garfinkel, accounts are only a partial representation of a complex reality and can only be appropriately interpreted if provider and recipient share a view of the underlying reality to which accounts refer. 'Trust' is then a matter of the confidence we have that we understand the underlying referents of others' accounts and thereby understand and anticipate their motives, behavior and (re)actions.

The approach to 'trust' taken here is based on Garfinkel's view. I make no attempt to precisely define or measure trust but attempt to 'surround it' through an example of redesign in the NHS in Scotland. This is a useful exercise, precisely because 'accounts' and 'accountability' are central to the redesign enterprise, and current debates center on the impact accountability has on trust. Service change also involves people reshaping relationships and a reappraisal of their place in a social system where they cannot be sure of others' assumptions and understandings of what is going on. The case of integrated health care informs this debate and provides a lens through which 'trust' can be made more visible.

6.1.3   Trust and Accountability in Health Care Organizations

The policies and practices of accountability are caught up in a number of tensions and paradoxes that may work against their intended effects. Most significantly, transparency and visible checks on practice may undermine, as well as foster confidence, because in human affairs rigorous checking is necessary only in situations of mistrust, and so introducing systems of public accountability sends the signal that there may be something not to be trusted (Strathearn 2000).

Current systems of accountability in U. K. health and other public services, such as education services, have far-reaching consequences for the way relationships are structured and trust built or eroded. Indeed some suggest that these systems amount to a cultural shift (Stathearn 2000). Established organizational structures of command are being dismantled and, in their stead, standards of service are set centrally, and staff are given the devolved power to police themselves against those standards. In other words, they are required to account for themselves. These systems of accountability are linked to objective and explicit standards and quality criteria so that subjective judgement is minimized and trust engendered (Dept. of Health 2000). Accounts are, however, never value free and 'naturally given' but human artefacts. They are social products with social consequences, which need to be managed to have the intended effects. This understanding allows us to ask a number of pertinent questions: Who are accounts produced by and for what purpose? Whose accounts come to be considered valid, and whose are not heard? Who acts on the accounts and to what end? And, crucially, who 'signs off' the final account and guarantees that the action, which flows from it, is for the recognized moral and social order of which Garfinkel speaks?

Organizations are big and opaque, and we tend to put our trust in people not systems (Calnan and Sandford 2004). 'Trust' is engendered or breached in face-to-face interactions, and the way that the organizational structures put in place to monitor these interactions impact on one-to-one interaction needs to be carefully considered (Dibben and Davies 2004). A tension thus emerges between the macroorganization of accountability on the one hand, and, on the other, the way this impacts on the relationships between individuals and between individuals and the organization.

This tension impacts in different ways in different settings (e.g., Mythen 2004). Local manifestations need to be understood and managed in order for systems of accountability to have the intended effect of building trust in and between members of health care organizations.

I present an ethnographic account of the way demands for accountability impact on integrated teams providing care for the elderly and for people with chronic and severe mental health problems. On the face of it, the teams appeared similar, each consisting of different professionals recruited from mainstream health and social services. These professionals were brought together in teams so they could more easily collaborate in the provision of flexible and timely care for individual clients by avoiding referral procedures embedded in their big parent organizations. On closer inspection, however, the teams, and the issues around trust and account-ability were very different.

6.2   TWO SETTINGS: INTEGRATED CARE AND INTEGRATED CARE PATHWAYS FOR OLDER PEOPLE AND PEOPLE WITH MENTAL HEALTH PROBLEMS IN SCOTLAND

Health services in developed economies are adapting to the current reali-ties of demographics and disease profiles by moving care for chronic and long-term conditions out of costly acute hospital facilities and into the com-munity. Closer alignment, or 'integration,' of health and social care is a prerequisite for these policies. In Scotland, legislation has been introduced to enable full integration of management and finances between health and social work organizations (Scottish Executive 2000). However, it appears that strategic direction at a national level does not always translate to effec-tive integration on the ground (Provan 1997), and issues remain around how to harmonize systems and procedures in two very different organiza-tions. Large-scale integration of core organizational components is pro-ceeding patchily and at a slow pace, but front-line integration is more easily accomplished through small-scale collaborative projects, such as teams providing services for a specific client group.

As a result of piecemeal development, the health and social care sector is fragmented; smaller services are introduced at different times and from different directions, often with short-term funding. Despite legislation, the fault lines between health and social work and between the different care professions are still visible. Staff are asked to relinquish their place in well-established organizational arrangements with clear and known benefits and disadvantages for something new and altogether unknown.

The part of the integrated landscape described here concerns commu-nity-based service provision for older people, to help them stay at home and thus avoid hospital admission or delayed discharges, and for people with mental health problems, to support them in the community and avoid crises that make admission or readmission to secondary care neces-sary. The service for older people consisted of teams of physiotherapists, occupational therapists, community nurses, social workers and home care managers. The mental health service teams were comprised of com-munity psychiatric nurses, occupational therapists and social workers. Staff were recruited or seconded into these teams from both health and social services.

There are numerous issues of 'trust' to be explored in these develop-ments. One issue of particular political concern is the way the fragmen-tation of services impacts on the safety of care. People with fluctuating mental health problems living outside the confines of institutions may be a risk to themselves and others; frail older people not looked after in hospital are vulnerable to accidents and relapses of illness, with potentially serious outcomes if undetected.

An Integrated Care Pathway (ICP; see e.g., De Luc 2000) is a tool that lends itself to creating coherence out of highly complex service provision. An ICP maps out the pathway of clinical and administrative events and activities for all professionals involved in care for a specific group of patients. The pathway outlines the routine tasks to be performed in chronological order in the patient's 'journey' through their care and specifies the input from different professionals in each task.

The concept of ICPs comes from engineering and was adopted by U.S. managed-care organizations as a way of monitoring costs of care and formalized operational procedures that involve multiagency work. The 1990s saw a surge in the use of ICPs in the United Kingdom. In 1998, approximately 250 NHS organizations were either developing or using care pathways in the United Kingdom (Currie 1999). Pathways are used for a number of purposes depending on the organization, need and patient population (De Luc 2000). For example, ICPs can be used as either a clinical management tool or a tool for clinical audit (Kitchiner et al. 1996). ICPs have been used to improve multidisciplinary documentation, communication and care planning (Higginson and Johnson 1997), as well as to improve systematic data collection and assessment of standards (Campbell et al. 1998).

An ICP is thus also a powerful tool of accountability. It divides complex care tasks into discrete 'chunks' that can be audited and allows variance from prescribed care to be tracked. ICPs thus exemplify well the many ways in which systems of accountability can impact on the day-to-day relationships that provide care and thereby affect the way 'trust' is fostered or eroded in everyday multidisciplinary work in fragmented and complex integrated settings.

6.3 METHODOLOGY: ETHNOGRAPHY IN ACTION RESEARCH

The research project on which this chapter draws was a national Scottish initiative termed 'Research-Based Development of Scottish Primary Care.' Collectively funded by all Scottish Primary Care Organizations, a team of researchers worked on projects identified by the Primary Care Organizations as high priority, as described above. One of these was 'Integration of health and social care for older people' and the other 'Integration of community-based services for people with chronic mental health problems.' Evaluations of integrated teams for care of older people, namely 'Rapid Response Teams,' in three Scottish Primary Care Organizations and integrated Community Mental Health Teams in one Primary Care Organization, became the focus of these two projects. In both settings, 'care pathways' were a conceptual and practical tool to structure and monitor the way professionals across health and social care worked together, but as I will explain, they were used differently.

The author led the project concerned with Rapid Response Teams, and a colleague led the project concerned with Community Mental Health Teams. As the two projects raised similar issues around integration, the accountability for integrated practice and the way accountability impacted on relationships between team members, and relationships between teams and the wider health and social care organizations to which they were accountable, we ran these two projects in parallel as a comparative case study.[1]

The collection and analysis of data was informed by the principles of ethnography. Data collection was shaped by three main interests: how the details of everyday practice were perceived by a range of team members and external stakeholders; team dynamics and how participants' perspectives were contested and negotiated in different situations; and how the pathway as an audit tool impacted on these dynamics.

We collected data through semistructured one-to-one and group interviews and from observations of team and project meetings. In the case of the Rapid Response Teams, we conducted baseline interviews with all teams and managers before we started our work with them, then follow-up interviews one year later. We conducted one group interview with all the Community Mental Health Teams and their managers.

We thus generated 'rich accounts' of team dynamics in relation to integration in the two settings and the impact of audit on these dynamics. Initial analysis identified key features of integration and audit across both projects. Further analysis proceeded according to the constant comparative method (Green 1998) and the principles of case study analysis (Mitchell 1983), where theoretical generalizations are made on the basis of comparison of the different *constellations* of trust in the two settings.

We aimed to work closely with the teams and their managers in both settings to help them identify key issues in the pathway, collect information regarding the way these impacted on the service and to interpret the information and draw practical implications. We thus became part of the process of constructing accounts and acting on them, and, to that extent, the impact we had on the teams became another source of data.

The researchers' relationships with the two services were, however, different. We formed collaborative relationships with the Rapid Response Teams and helped them use the pathway methodology to achieve recognition and increased security within their parent health and social service organizations. The Community Mental Health Teams, on the other hand, resisted a management-led introduction of a formal ICP and were wary of our role in this process. They were unsure if we were an instrument of management control or facilitators of an implementation strategy that took teams' concerns into account.

Trust, in the sense of a shared understanding between the researchers and the researched about the purpose of the enterprise, is profoundly implicated in research, both in terms of production of 'trustworthy' accounts and in the appropriate interpretation of the accounts offered. There was a high degree of trust between the researchers and the Rapid Response Teams, because we had confidence that we shared an understanding of integration and its key issues in this setting. There was a lack of trust between the researchers and the Community Mental Health Teams, because the teams were unsure of our agenda, and we, as researchers, were not confident that the teams fully shared their understanding with us, which limited our interpretation of teams' accounts.

The Community Mental Health Teams' caution was, perhaps, warranted in the end. Although the research team was sent in by the Primary Care Organizations to facilitate team work and generate its accounts—and so in theory could have helped build the systems of communication generating trust—in practice, the research team itself may have become part of the problem of fragmented systems of accountability in a fragmented service system. We were a small research project introduced through a route that few people understood, and our role was not always clear. By the time we had established relationships with the teams and their managers, the NHS in Scotland had been reorganized, and the Primary Care Organizations, who were our funders and champions, disappeared. The project was then disbanded.

6.4   THE TEAMS: CARE OF OLDER PEOPLE AND MENTAL HEALTH TEAMS COMPARED

We worked with Rapid Response Teams for care of the elderly in three areas (areas A, B and C) and five Community Mental Health Teams in one area. An analysis of the team dynamics and the impact of pathways on teams' work has been presented elsewhere (Rees et al. 2004; Huby and Rees 2005). Here I present a short summary of the factors that structured teamwork in the two services and outline their implications for teamwork and accountability.

Rapid Response Teams were established following a report about integration of health and social care for the elderly that emphasized the need to reduce pressure on acute care and to react to care needs of older people more quickly than the procedures of mainstream health and social work organizations allowed (Scottish Executive 2000). Teams were set up in different ways in different localities, though they had certain features in common.

Team members relinquished their place within their old organization or profession when they became Rapid Response staff, and team members from all the areas said that they had been warned by colleagues against applying for these jobs because they would lose professional status, credibility and security. All team members said they felt deskilled in terms of the knowledge required for mainstream posts, and the longer they remained in the teams, the more uncertain they felt their positions in mainstream services became.

The management arrangements were fragmented. Teams were managed by representatives from both health and social care, whose workload left little time for development of the service. Added complexities stemmed from the number of different stakeholders within each organization, reflecting the multiprofessional nature of the teams. In addition to everyday operational managers, team members needed supervision from their own professions, because there is no recognized 'profession' of Rapid Response Teams. These arrangements resulted in a curious mix of overmanagement by a range of stakeholders, on the one hand, and a lack of management, in terms of lack of clear decision-making structures and strategic direction, on the other.

In the space created by lack of clear line management, teams had a large degree of freedom to do things their own way and to find their own solutions to problems. The fact that teams' involvement with their clients was time-limited, and the clients were discharged back into mainstream care after a set period, made it possible to circumscribe this space. Teams learned to with-hold problems and issues from supervisors and managers, because small and practical problems could be exacerbated if they became the object of contest between stakeholders. At the time of our involvement with the three teams, the services were 'pilot' projects with insecure funding, and the shared lack of security forged additional bonds of solidarity between team members.

In summary, then, the Rapid Response Teams at the time sat rather uneasily between mainstream health and social care organizations. Joining a team meant breaking loose from a well-defined place in a well-established system and quickly forging new relationships in teams which had to rely on their own resources to make the service work.

Community Mental Health Teams (CMHTs), by contrast, have a longer history than Rapid Response Teams and have emerged more 'organically.' The five Community Mental Health teams taking part in this project grew out of a five-year process of formalization of the Community Mental Health Service, as institutional care for people with mental health problems was gradually replaced by care in the community. Three of the teams grew out of informal joint working arrangements that had developed over a long time, and the remaining two were set up from scratch. As part of this process, teams were co-located and team leaders appointed. This picture is reflected across the United Kingdom, with teams often developing locally in an informal manner based on historical contextual factors such as existing working relationships between individual professionals (Peck and Parker 1998). More recently CMHTs have been formed strategically. The formation over time of the teams meant that they represented less of a sudden break from members' previous working arrangements than was the case for Rapid Response Teams.

Another key difference was the nature of the work: Rapid Response Teams worked with patients on a time-limited basis, with a specific goal.

They took full responsibility for the patient during that time, but this responsibility was time-limited. Managing chronic mental health problems in the community is an altogether different challenge. Care is not time-limited but an ongoing commitment that requires constant liaison with other care providers. People's health improves or deteriorates for reasons outside care workers' control and in ways which take no account of fluctuations in teams' resources and responsibilities. As I will demonstrate, being 'swamped' was, therefore, a danger against which team members sought to protect themselves.

Protection came in large part from the professional boundaries of the 'parent' professions and health and social work organizations. These boundaries were reinforced by employment arrangements, which were different from those of the Rapid Response Teams. The teams were formed from multidisciplinary professionals working as part of and, paid by, mainstream health and social work organizations. Social workers in particular had duties outside the teams, which could take substantial amounts of time away from their work as team members. Other professionals were therefore reluctant to share the team's social work tasks because they could not rely on social workers returning the favor.

Dedicated management resources had been put in place. Each team had a team leader, and the service was in addition managed by one manager from health and one from social work. The team leaders in particular were in a difficult position. Their job was to ensure joint working within teams, but they had little power to break down the professional boundaries team members brought with them into the teams.

Community Mental Health Teams, then, were more firmly lodged within the organizational structures of mainstream health and social work. Team members looked to the professional boundaries of the 'old' order to protect themselves from the demands of the service. This pulled team members away from the teams and from reliance on their team colleagues.

6.5   TRUST AND ACCOUNTABILITY

The way the two services developed, and the conditions of the service, produced very different kinds of teams, with very different receptiveness to accountability. The Rapid Response Teams developed a highly integrated service for which they were keen to account in order to secure a future for the service. In contrast, for Community Mental Health Teams, the organization of the service made it more difficult to become fully integrated. Moreover, a formal system of accountability for integration was put in place, but it proved difficult to provide the required accounts

In the following section I present a picture of the dynamics of teamwork in the two services and how the systems of accountability introduced impacted on these relations.

6.5.1   Rapid Response Teams

The history of these teams produced an 'us versus the world' attitude, which was highly conducive to integration and team cohesiveness.

> **Nurse:** But we're not completely protective of our roles. Like I don't think like 'I'm a nurse and you're not a nurse and you're not doing that 'and we don't think like 'you're not doing social work stuff.' We're quite happy to blur, we quite like, you know, makes it more interesting when we're doing things that we haven't done. But I think further up it's to do with budgets and to do with territories and whatever. There's no agreement and then that affects us because they all sort of make the rules for their little area.

> **Interviewer:** Just conflicting information?

> **Nurse:** Yeah, changing all the time.

> **Social worker:** And there's confusion and conflict because some people are very happy for us to be pragmatic and to find our ways round and sort of blur things and learn from each other on a hands-on basis and other people aren't. (Team interview, Area A, Oct. 2002).

For example, quick and timely access to occupational therapy (OT) equipment and adaptations was an issue for teams in all areas. Occupational therapists were unhappy about letting outsiders request and access equipment they felt only trained OTs could use because of issues around accountability for safety and cost. Teams handled this by working together to find ways around the problems. In Area A an OT set up training for non-OTs in the safe management of basic equipment, and this was accepted by the OT department as sufficient.

Working together in this way created ownership and pride in the service:

> **Nurse:** We can sort things out between ourselves to a very large extent and I mean there's obviously things we don't manage to, but I think that's the natural, you know, that's to be expected. I think it would be unrealistic not to have some irresolvable issues but I do think to a large extent there's a lot of things that we just work together with.

> **Interviewer:** So with the management issue whilst it clearly does have some implications on, at some level in the way that you work, there's quite a lot of positive aspects of it as well.

> **All:** Yeah! (Interview, Team 3, Area B, Oct. 2002).

The daily contact meant that an understanding built up within the teams about what the service was about.

Nurse: And I think at the end of the day the patients and family benefit more.

Interviewer: In what way do you think they benefit?

Nurse: I just think things don't get missed, things don't, you know, it's not for the sake of things getting missed but I just think that things can get identified quicker so they get implemented quicker, services get put in quicker. I mean they go out with a fractured hip but you've also sorted their hearing, you know, they've got oral thrush, you've identified that they've got incontinence. Now these things would be missed, I know they would be missed at ward level.

Physiotherapist: Things like the community alarm and the services and then social work. (Interview, Team 1, Area A, Nov. 2003).

Team members learned about each others' skills, roles and responsibilities, and they could exchange roles to a large extent. For example, an OT was happy for a social worker or a nurse to check equipment and had confidence in a non-OT colleague's recommendations about care equipment. Nurses could request daily domestic help directly from the social work home care manager without this request being checked. However, although teams had a clear account of their work and its value, it was not clear to them who was there to listen to their account or indeed what accounts potential audiences were interested in. Issues of accountability mirrored the fragmentation of management: They were not clear, and there was no consensus regarding what the teams were accountable for.

Accountability

The bottom line in terms of accountability was proving that the teams reduced pressure on acute services by bringing down the number of delayed discharges and emergency hospital admissions of older people. To this end, teams provided regular returns to The Scottish Executive Health Department[2], in terms of 'saved bed days' and to the Scottish Executive Social Work Department, in terms of numbers of patients seen. The managers who were accountable for the funding privileged these returns.

There was no feedback on this information from funders, and teams did not know what was done with the data. Neither was it known whether the Scottish Executive Social Work and Health departments coordinated the analysis and interpretation of the returns. In both areas, there was a sense of sending data off as a matter of administrative routine into a system over which nobody had an overview and from which no feedback was provided.

All teams routinely collected a range of data on their activity. Routine databases were big and somewhat unwieldy. Often, columns were added as a result of outside agencies requesting data. Teams also collected data which they thought showed the value of their service better than the saved bed days returns. However, apart from the saved bed days returns and number of clients seen, data were never systematically analyzed, shared and discussed among teams and their many stakeholders.

> **Occupational Therapist:** . . . and in terms of how you measure like the [saved bed] days and things like that, although, we try but the likes of working in the team and things like that, it's a very difficult thing we've never come up with . . . We know we do it and we know it makes a difference because we know that when we see patients we're able to access each other and each others services very rapidly and very effectively but we don't know how to record it in a way, you know, that makes it look like we're actually achieving anything different from normal services. (Interview, Team 1, Area B, Oct. 2002).

There was therefore a strong wish to make visible what the teams themselves saw as a valuable part of their service and the effect that had on the quality of the care they provided.

> **Interviewer:** What is it that you actually want to achieve by carrying out this process [of evaluation]?
>
> **Physiotherapist:** I suppose as I say basically at the end of the day it's being able to achieve effective care.
>
> **Nurse:** To be able to prove that it's working from the evaluation.
>
> **Physiotherapist:** Yes, what we're doing is saying yes we have succeeded, that we have kept X number of patients out of hospital beds, successfully and happily.
>
> **Nurse:** And improved and done it. They are better off for being through the Rapid Response Team not worse off.
>
> **Physiotherapist:** And that we have improved the situation.
>
> **Nurse:** We're not just doing it because this is what the Scottish Executive wants, it's actually worth doing it. (Interview, Team 1, Area B, Oct. 2002).

Rapid Response teams, then, were made accountable for aspects of the service that they did not see as the most important, by using data that they considered unreliable, which was provided to an organization that they did not understand. They had no clear idea of how they fitted in and whether their place was secure. They had little confidence in the wider 'system' of budgets and 'territories' in which the team was placed; instead they focused on building trust within the team and in a way of working together that they believed worked for patients and from which they derived great personal satisfaction.

Input from Evaluation Project

Researchers from the evaluation project worked with the teams to construct reliable accounts of the service in their own terms. We helped teams construct routine databases that picked up the aspects they believed were important. Database construction allowed them to monitor their impact in these areas. We also provided them with training in qualitative audit methods that allowed for the 'softer' aspects of the service to be documented (Rees, Edmunds and Huby 2005). We ran joint workshops where teams from different areas came together and learned from each other.

The aim of this input was twofold: to help teams build evaluation reports that provided meaningful accounts of the service from the teams' point of view and to help them use the evaluation to improve communication about the service between and within the organizations involved. We were successful on both counts. Teams took to the self-auditing with enthusiasm and commitment. We also held several successful meetings and seminars where we pulled in representatives from the teams' organizations and the Scottish Executive Health Department to facilitate discussion on the kinds of information about the service that was relevant and useful and how it could be shared.

However, particularly in Area A, there was a rapid turnover of personnel in teams, and the organization of the service went through several permutations. It was difficult therefore to sustain the engagement over time. More importantly, our research team was also an impermanent feature of the integrated care landscape. We were only in operation for three years and effective in this setting for only one of those.

6.5.2   Community Mental Health Teams

Whereas, the Rapid Response Teams developed role blurring and integration of tasks within teams as a way of working, CMHTs relied on professional boundaries to a much greater extent.

> **Community Psychiatric Nurse:** Because that's people, obviously, for any worker, and it doesn't matter if its mental health or where it is, you've got to have some boundaries. You set yourself some boundaries

to avoid getting swamped. And it's only when you begin to trust your colleagues from different disciplines that you will relax those a bit and come and go with people.

Interviewer: Uh huh.

Community Psychiatric Nurse: Erm, that maybe sounds a bit negative but I think that is a personal survival thing for anyone working in health or social services, because we all have the potential to get swamped . . .

Interviewer: Uh huh.

Community Psychiatric Nurse: Because there is lots of work to do.

Interviewer: Yeah.

Community Psychiatric Nurse: And it doesn't really have an ending. (Interview, Team 2, Dec. 2002).

Some role blurring was necessary for the team to function as intended. This principle was embedded in the role of a 'key worker' whose duty it was to ensure that appropriate care was set up and coordinated. This was a social worker responsibility in the 'old' order of health and social care. In the team, however, it made some sense for the team member in closest contact with the client to take this task on. A duty linked to the key worker function was to do the paperwork needed to set up a care package, and this was time consuming.

This discussion in one of the team interviews illustrates particularly well resistance to the idea of full integration in terms of role blurring and sharing of the care package task, and it also suggests some of the interprofessional dynamics at play.

Social Worker: . . . . it's to do with joint working and it's to do with what joint working means, I mean I'm supposed to hold, or to joint work all care packages. That's the view because that's what my predecessor did and that's what's the traditional view [of] social work in this team, or at least that's part of the social work role. . . . well why do I need to do that? Why is that part of the social work role? Because it's an admin function . . . . And the key worker is the person who knows the client, the key person is the person who has regular contact with the carers probably, if having regular contact with the client then there's no reason, in my view, why, and it seems to make for an enormous amount of duplication for the social worker, for one, even if it's not the social worker, for anybody on the team to have to go to the key worker and find out lots of things in order to complete forms.

Community Psychiatric Nurse: Who's going to do what. . . . Because as the OT says, if nobody's got specific roles then what do we do in the team?. . . . Because there's things that only myself and other CPNs can do, like give injections. . . . There's things that only the OTs qualified in, which is the occupational therapy assessments and certain programs that he's you know, brilliant at . . . Erm so we've got to kind of look at, well if you're not doing this and that's what you're here for, then what's—then what are you here for kind of thing?

Social Worker: Yeah I mean we we've all got specific areas that nobody else can do and you know, sort of mental health legislation would be you know, the, social work [role] which you know take up an awful, well quite a lot of time, erm you know that's that's the social work thing, erm in terms of specifics that nobody else can do. Erm but what I'll debate about of course is care packages which . . .

Community Psychiatric Nurse: It's what it comes down to . . .

Social Worker: Which I mean . . .

Community Psychiatric Nurse: "Nobody's trained in, is that right? Nobody, you're not trained to do that either, are you?" (Interview, Team 2, Dec. 2002).

Accountability

In order to strengthen multidisciplinary working within the teams, two managers—one from the primary Care NHS Trust and one from the social work department—developed an Integrated Care Pathway (ICP) for implementation within all teams which formalized, documented and made explicit and auditable collaboration and cooperation between different professionals within the teams.

In the area concerned, the ICP was a novel idea, because it brought together the paperwork and systems used by social work and health care into one system. The ICP thus structured collaborative practices and required that this be documented and made explicit for the purpose of audit and continuous improvement.

The teams, for their part, were unanimous about the potential benefits of the ICP.

Team Member 1:[3] We have to have the right support, it can only enhance what we do and it will make us, record and document work that is already being done and things that are already happening and its just going to make it much more easily identified, who's doing what, where the key packages are, what's happening, when it's going to be, and who is going to do it? It all happens just now, it's all done, but it's held by various people and it's brought to the team at different times, and it's just going to collate all that information together.

Team Member 2: And it will definitely improve our kind of work with users and carers, definitely formalizing that [. . .]

Team Member 3: "It will make it very clear what it is that we're doing and also make it very clear what it is we're not doing. (Interview, Team 1, Jan. 2003).

In spite of a clear understanding of potential benefits, however, the teams resisted the implementation of the ICP. In interviews they quoted several reasons, which all had to do with lack of ownership of the new systems that had been put in place:

Team Member 1: This does take a lot of time effort and energy to put this, to change over, and we could all see that it, it could be really beneficial, as we can see, where we would like to be. And we can see where we are now and we have no idea how to get there, you know. And it doesn't seem to me like there's been an awful lot of time or effort put in supporting people to get to that stage. There was quite a lot of effort put in to tell us about the ICP, and how it should work, and what all the paperwork was about. But there was, I don't think enough put in to help people get there.

Team Member 2: The feeling I had was there was an awful lot of work to be put in, put in initially, from the paperwork point of view. And they've all seemed to fade away, I don't know it's sort of tailed off somehow (laughter).

Team Member 3: As long as it doesn't go the way that other things have gone like care programming and things like that, which were well funded, and all this sort of buzz went on round about them. And then over the years the funding was kind of reduced and coordinators.

Team Member 1: The coordinator had disappeared.

Team Member 3: (cont.) taken away to do other things and it imploded. . . . And the big danger with ICP is that it could do the same thing quite easily. Because once the initial momentum goes and you know people like yourselves stop coming to evaluate it, and it's not trendy anymore with the Scottish Office. The danger is that it'll, it'll die a death.

Team Member 1: So we won't worry about it too much, there'll be something else.

Team Member 3: I think there's a danger in that (Interview Team 1, Jan. 2003).

The Community Mental Health Teams were clearly disenchanted with the ICP and had no confidence in the power of their managers and the organizations they represented to make them accountable for the way they worked within the teams.

Role of the Evaluation Project

The evaluation project offered to work with the teams to identify what kind of support was needed to implement the ICP and how the ICP itself had to change to better reflect the reality of teamwork. The approach suggested was the same one successfully adopted with the Rapid Response Teams, namely to help the teams construct an account of the service which was meaningful to them. This was, however, not taken up and the teams resisted our involvement as they resisted the ICP itself.

The lack of confidence these teams had in the researchers meant that we cannot be sure we fully appreciated the underlying understanding teams had of integration, its incentives and disincentives and why they did not want to account for their practice. The accounts generated through the evaluation thus give an incomplete picture of reasons behind the teams' resistance. Did they resist being made accountable because integrated practice was difficult in their circumstances, or did they make integration and accountability look difficult because they were resisting? Either way, we were not let into their confidence and were unable to help them share their views within the organization and facilitate a common understanding.

6.6   DISCUSSION

'Trust' is not an either–or phenomenon but a dynamic dimension of social life, and it can only be understood in context. It overlaps with faith, commitment, confidence and reliance, and I have not tried to distinguish between them. Rather, 'trust' is defined broadly as people's reason to take for granted a certain moral and social order and their place in it (Garfinkel 1967). The social order is a fine-meshed fabric held together by checks and balances of a range of dimensions: loyalty and disloyalty, intimacy and distance, reliance and deceit. In order to function, we need a reason to trust that our overall understanding of the social terrain holds true. We also need to know that our understanding and interests are at the very least noted but preferably also shared and respected by others. It is this overall understanding that is easily undermined in a situation of organizational change such as the emergence of the intermediate or integrated care sector, because it is easy to lose social bearings.

This chapter builds up an account of teams which ostensibly worked to the same aims and philosophy but in which circumstances shaped the social order of their practice in very different ways and hence created different conditions for production of trust within the teams. Rapid Response staff looked to the teams for a shared understanding and hence trust. Community Mental Health Team members, on the other hand, turned to their 'parent' organizations and professions for a place they could trust. They brought their professional and organizational boundaries into the teams to protect them from the danger inherent in the potentially unlimited demands of their client group.

Issues around accountability were, however, similar. Both Rapid Response Teams and Community Mental Health Teams were asked to account for themselves; and the circumstances around this duty eroded, rather than engendered, trust. Rapid Response Teams were eager to account for what they saw as good practice in integrated care, and for them the integrated pathway concept became an instrument of empowerment and a vehicle for their accounts of themselves. However, nobody asked for such accounts. Instead, they were asked to submit accounts about an aspect of the service they did not consider the most important with information they deemed unreliable. The Community Mental Health Teams for their part resisted being made accountable at all, for a number of reasons. The teams were struggling to work in an integrated way in the first place, something that auditing of the ICP could only serve to highlight. Moreover, the teams did not feel involved in and informed about the implementation of the ICP. Importantly, neither service had reason to be confident and clear about the use to which their accounts would be put. Indeed, they had no reason to believe that their accounts would be used at all.

A range of factors was involved in the production of trust in the process of redesign and organizational change described here. Clear social boundaries delineating where trust can be placed is important. The opportunity for teams to account for themselves and claim a place and role in the setting, which was known and understood both by the team and other important stakeholders, was another. The circumstances around the sharing of these accounts, or rather the fact that they were not shared, was however a crucial element in the way they failed to generate trust.

It is precisely the negotiation around accounts that produces a shared understanding of the new social order and individual workers' place in it. In both cases this negotiation was lacking because the relationships were not in place. The balance between internal autonomy of teams and mechanisms of external control that can link the teams to the wider sector of integrated care—and be a vehicle for the sharing and negotiation of accounts—is a particularly important issue here. For the Rapid Response Teams and the Community Mental Health Teams, this balance was not achieved. As a result, in neither case did the notion of a pathway underpin the development of a social order around integration, which was based on trust.

6.7 PRACTICAL IMPLICATIONS

Systems of accountability such as ICPs can be rather blunt instruments for the engineering of delicate social processes. In spite of the intention to produce trust through greater transparency, their introduction alone will clearly not guarantee trust in the kind of settings described here. The conditions in which accountability systems are introduced and the way they are used are as, or more, important than their technicalities (Walsh and Freeman 2002). In the right conditions they can no doubt underpin and strengthen already existing trust. They can, however, also undermine and erode trust, and it is unlikely that systems of accountability themselves can engender trust where none exists in the first place.

The examples presented here suggest that accountability can easily become meaningless if accounts become separated from human interaction. For accountability to foster trust, relationships that embed the production and interpretation of accounts in a known and shared social order must be in place.

A good pathway will provide the information needed for good management, but it is no substitute for a personal understanding of the setting and footwork undertaken to bring people on board and structure a process of negotiation about the ideal and the feasible in service reorganization. The way different stakeholders are brought into these negotiations will be key to the production of trust. Squaring this circle is a challenge in the case of intermediate or integrated care, because the sector is complex and shifting, with new projects coming in and existing services changing function and role. Pockets of good practice are possible to achieve, but linking the many small initiatives into something coherent and trusted may be another matter.

ACKNOWLEDGMENTS

Thanks to the teams and their managers for facilitating the studies and to Gwyneth Rees for collaboration on the project.

NOTES

1. This study was carried out in 2002. There have been further changes in the organisation of health and social care since then, but this research focuses on the implications arising from reorganisation at that particular stage.
2. The Scottish Regional Government Health Department.
3. Profession of respondent is not given in this quote as it is not relevant to the data presented.

6.9 REFERENCES

Beck, U. 1992. *Risk Society: Towards a New Modernity*. London: Routledge.

Calnan, M., and E. Sandford. 2004. Public trust in health care: The system or the doctor? *Quality and Safety in Health Care* 13 (2): 92–97.

Campbell, H., R. Hotchkiss, N. Bradshaw, and M. Porteous. 1998. Integrated care pathways. *British Medical Journal* 316: 133–137.

Checkland, K., M. Marshall, and S. Harrison. 2004. Rethinking accountability; trust versus confidence in medical practice. *Quality and Safety in Health Care* 13 (2): 130–135.

Currie, L. 1999. Researching care pathway development in the United Kingdom: Stage 1. *Nursing Times Research* 4: 378–382.

Davies, H. 1999. Falling public trust in health services. *Journal of Health Services Research and Policy* 14: 193–194.

De Luc, K. 2000. Care pathways: An evaluation of their effectiveness. *Journal of Advanced Nursing* 32 (2): 485–496.

Department of Health. 1998. *The New NHS Modern and Dependable: A National Framework for Assessing Performance*. NHS Executive.

Dibben, M. R., and H. Davies. 2004. Trustworthy doctors in confidence building stems. *Quality and Safety in Health Care* 13 (2): 88–89.

Garfinkel, H. 1967. *Studies in Ethnomethodology*. Englewood Cliffs: Prentice-Hall [paperback edition].

Green, J. 1998. Commentary: Grounded theory and the constant comparative method. *British Medical Journal* 316: 1064–1065.

Higginson, A., and S. Johnson. 1997. Pathways bridging the acute/community interface. In *Pathways of Care,* ed. S. Johnson, 133–149. Oxford: Blackwell Science.

Huby, G., and G. Rees. 2005. The effectiveness of Quality Improvement Tools: Joint working in integrated community teams. *International Journal of Quality in Health Care* 17 (1): 53–58.

Kitchiner, D., C. Davidson, and P. Bunred. 1996. Integrated Care Pathways: Effective tools for continuous evaluation of clinical practice. *Journal of Evaluation in Clinical Practice* 2: 65–69.

Luhmann, N. 1979. *Trust and Power*. New York: Wiley.

Mitchell, J. C. 1983. Case and situation analysis. *Social Review* 31: 187–211.

Mythen, G. 2004. *Ulrich Beck: A Critical Introduction to the Risk Society*. Pluto Press: London: Sterling VA.

Peck, Parker E. 1998. Mental Health in the NHS: Policy and Practice 1997–1998. *Journal of Mental Health* 7: 241–260.

Provan, G. K. 1997. Services integration for vulnerable populations: Lessons from community mental health. *Family & Community Health* 19 (4): 19–30.

Rees, G., G. Huby, L. McDade, and L. McKechnie. 2004. Joint working in community mental health teams: Implementation of an Integrated Care Pathway. *Journal of Health and Social Care in the Community* 12 (6): 527–536.

Rees, G., S. Edmunds, and G. Huby. 2005. Evaluation and development of integrated teams: The use of Significant Event Analysis. *Journal of Interprofessional Care* 19 (2): 125–136.

Rowe, R., and M. Calnan. 2006. Trust relations in health care: Developing a theoretical framework for the 'new' NHS. *Journal of Health Care Organization and Management* 20 (5): 376–396.

Scottish Executive. 2000. *Report of the Joint Future Group*. Edinburgh: Scottish Executive.

Strathearn, M., ed. 2002. *Audit Cultures: Anthropological Studies in Accountability, Ethics and the Academy*. London: Routledge.

Walsh, K., and T. Freeman. 2002. Effectiveness of quality improvement: Learning from evaluations. *Quality and Safety in Health Care* 11 (1): 85–87.

7 Trust and Asymmetry in General Practitioner–Patient Relationships in the United Kingdom

Bruce Guthrie

7.1 BACKGROUND

High-profile cases of system or individual failure are widely perceived as eroding public and patient faith in medicine (Davies 1999; Mechanic 1996), although evidence for this from surveys of patients and the public is weak at best (Calnan and Sanford 2004; Van der Schee, Groenewegen and Friele 2006). Regulatory reform has sought to reduce the risk of such failures by increasing external measurement and oversight of medical practice. Improving patient and public trust in health care is a central aim of such reform (Secretary of State for Health 2007), although such an expansion of the 'audit society' (Power 2003) itself has been argued to reduce trust (O'Neill 2002; Strathern 2000). One response from organized medicine has been to reaffirm the importance of 'professionalism' (Jacobs 2005; Rosen and Dewar 2004), by promoting new models of the social contract between doctors and society:

> "Professionalism is the basis of medicine's contract with society. It demands placing the interests of patients above those of the physician, setting and maintaining standards of competence and integrity, and providing expert advice to society on matters of health. . . . Essential to this contract is public trust in physicians, which depends on the integrity of both individual physicians and the whole profession." (ABIM Foundation et al. 2002, 244).

Trust is therefore central to current claims by doctors to the privileges of professional status and autonomy (Kao et al. 1998). However, doctors rarely define what they mean by trust or consider it in the wider context of doctor–patient relationships. This chapter examines trust in the relationship between general practitioners (GPs)[1] and patients.

7.1.1 What is Trust?

Trust has many definitions, but Davies proposes that:

'All embody the notion of expectations: expectations by the public that healthcare providers will demonstrate knowledge, skill and competence; further expectations too that they will behave as true agents (that is in the patient's best interests) and with beneficence, fairness and integrity. It is these collective expectations that form the basis of trust.' (Davies 1999, 193).

Optimistic collective expectations are the basis of 'social' or 'systems' trust in the institutions of medicine, nursing, hospitals, and the National Health Service (NHS), in particular hospitals or practices, or in doctors in general (Fugelli 2001; Hall et al. 2001; Pearson and Raeke 2000). Social trust frames trust in particular doctors, as it allows a patient to initially trust individuals about whom they know little except that they are doctors (Dibben and Davies 2004; Hall et al. 2001). Similarly, collective expectations are modified by patients' experience of care (Keating et al. 2002), leading to less blind 'interpersonal' trust in (or mistrust of) particular doctors. Expectations of particular doctors are partly based on their communication skills in individual consultations (Hall et al. 2001; Mechanic and Meyer 2000) but more strongly on experience over repeated consultation, which creates a deeper relationship (Burkitt-Wright, Holcombe and Salmon 2004; Thorne and Robinson 1989). Interpersonal trust is often said to be based on patients' judgments about technical competence (medical expertise), interpersonal competence (communication, compassion, care), and agency (the belief that the doctor is committed to the patient's best interests) (Goudge and Gilson 2005; Hall et al. 2001; Thom and Campbell 1997). However, in practice patients appear to judge technical competence largely on the basis of interpersonal cues between themselves and health professionals (Burkitt-Wright, Holcombe and Salmon 2004; Mechanic and Meyer 2000; Thom and Campbell 1997).

Accounts of trust often overemphasize the cognitive bases of trust, focusing on the 'good reasons' that people give for trusting (Möllering 2001). Trust may also be accredited with a strong affective component that goes beyond cognitive judgments and distinguishes it from other kinds of expectations, such as reliance. We may all expect our cars to start in the morning but are merely annoyed if our expectations of reliability are not met. In contrast, a breach of trust is emotionally painful, and therefore perceived as a betrayal (Rogers 2002). From this perspective, trust always involves a 'leap of faith' in which uncertainties about the behavior of others and the future are suspended. Individuals interpret their act of trusting in terms of good reasons for making such a leap, but these good reasons are only weakly related to the suspension required because there are usually other good reasons not to trust (Brownlie and Howson 2005; Möllering 2001). Indeed, trust would not be necessary if there were no uncertainty.

Trust therefore exists within relationships and is voluntarily granted by a person in a vulnerable situation because of expectations about the trusted person's or institution's motives and future actions (Gilson 2006). Trust matters because it allows all of us to function without constant suspicion and checking, thereby underpinning social capital (Ahern and Hendryx 2003). In healthcare, trust may also have instrumental benefits, as it is associated with greater disclosure of relevant, sensitive information and greater adherence to medical advice (Thom, Hall and Pawlson 2004).

7.1.2   What is the Role of the Patient?

In the medical literature on trust, both social and interpersonal trust are generally framed in terms of the public and patients as trusting (or not) and medicine and doctors as trustworthy (or not). External regulation and management are often cast as threats to trust and therefore to access and effectiveness (Kao et al. 1998; Mechanic 1996). Consequently, measures of trust are largely designed to allow patients to quantify trust in particular professionals, hospitals or insurers, or in professions, institutions, or health systems more generally (Calnan and Sanford 2004; Hall et al. 2002). Less attention is paid to the idea of doctors trusting patients, despite the importance ascribed to mutual doctor–patient relationships and patients' expertise in self-management (Tuckett 1985; RCGP 2004; RCGP et al. 2001; Department of Health 2006). Doctors are likely to form expectations of future behavior by patients in situations where care is for chronic disease or where long-term relationships are common, both of which particularly apply to general practice (RCGP 2004; RCGP et al. 2001). However, these expectations are not usually framed in terms of trust. The rationale for this is that doctors are not seen as vulnerable in the way that patients are and so do not have to form trusting expectations of future behaviour from patients (Hall et al. 2001). From this perspective, even if doctors rely on patients to tell the truth and follow medical advice, they do not usually feel betrayed if patients do not.

In contrast, Rogers (2002) argues that respect for patient autonomy requires doctors to trust patients or at least to 'aspire to trust and to adopt a trusting attitude' (2002, 79) because to do otherwise is to reject the validity of patient experience and suffering, particularly where existing medical models of disease are unhelpful. Trusting in this way may leave the doctor vulnerable if the patient is deceiving them (as may happen where addictive drugs are being prescribed or access to welfare benefits is at stake) and open to feelings of betrayal (Rogers 2002). Others have argued that if patients are to play an active role in patient safety, for example by checking their treatments, then health care professionals will have to trust patients not to apportion blame unfairly or be litigious in their response to safety problems (Entwistle and Quick 2006). This extends the potential scope of trust in patients to areas of knowledge and expertise over which doctors claim professional jurisdiction (Abbott 1988).

Reflecting this perspective, empirical work on trust in professional–patient relationships has focused on patient or public trust in professionals and institutions (Brownlie and Howson 2005; Calnan and Sanford 2004; Mechanic and Meyer 2000; Thom and Campbell 1997). A partial exception is Thorne and Robinson's (1989) longitudinal study of the experiences of patients affected by Chronic disease. They found that initial 'naïve trust' of patients in professionals gives way to 'disenchantment' as patients face the limitations of medical care and then to various forms of 'guarded alliance.' In the most mutual form of guarded alliance, doctors trusting patients' expertise in understanding and managing their chronic disease helped facilitate self-management and strengthened patients' trust in doctors. In order to further examine trust in the relationship between general practitioners and patients, this chapter now draws on data from interviews with sixteen GPs and thirty-two patients, conducted as part of a study that examined what GPs and patients valued about U.K. general practice. The analysis presented here focuses on how GPs and patients talked about trust, and discusses the taken-for-granted assumptions about trust within these accounts.

7.2   METHODOLOGY

The research was conducted from the perspective of 'subtle realism' (Hammersley 1992). This is a perspective where it is assumed we can be reasonably confident, but never certain, about the validity of knowledge claims. It assumes that there is a reality independent of claims made about it and that the validity of knowledge depends on its correspondence to this reality. The aim of social research is to represent this reality as far as possible. Representation is always from some point of view that emphasizes some aspects of reality over others. To choose a method is to choose a point of view, and there can be 'multiple, non-contradictory and valid descriptions and explanations of the same phenomenon' (Hammersley 1992, 51). Research is, therefore, an interpretive undertaking, where data are constructed jointly by the researcher and the researched in the social context within which the research is embedded. This subtle realism represents a weak form of social constructionism, yet there is still assumed to be some correspondence to an underlying, albeit not completely knowable, reality (Seale 1999).

From this perspective, all interview data are jointly created in the social interaction between interviewer and interviewee (Seale 1999). Interview data are never a description of the facts of the topic at hand but, rather, are an account whose form and content are shaped by the context of the interview. For instance, in this study, a particular issue is that participants knew that the interviewer—myself—was also a GP. A likely impact of this knowledge on the GP interviews is that they may have been more willing to make more negative judgments of patient behavior than if interviewed by a nonclinician (Chew-Graham, May and Perry 2002). In contrast, interviewed patients are likely to have been less critical of doctors in general (in which case the data will overstate the strength of 'social' trust in doctors) and of particular doctors (in which case the data will understate the degree to which patients mistrust some or all of the GPs they know). Thus, having a medical interviewer may make it less likely that in-depth accounts of patient mistrust and their strategies of verification in the development of trust will be revealed. The analysis should, therefore, be read with this in mind.

The study was approved by an NHS Research Ethics Committee in Scotland, and data collection and analysis have been described elsewhere (Guthrie and Wyke 2006). In brief, an initial pilot study of a convenience sample of six GPs and four patients was used to refine the study questions and topic guide. The main study used purposive sampling to ensure heterogeneity of participants. Ten GPs were recruited from practices varying in size and the socioeconomic deprivation of the populations they served. Each GP recruited three patients, two with chronic disease (diabetes and high blood pressure) and one without any major chronic disease. To avoid only recruiting patients that GPs had close relationships with, GPs were asked to recruit at least one person with chronic disease that they *knew well* and one person they *had some knowledge of but would not say they knew well*. Patients recruited varied in their use of general practice (from 0–20 consultations in the previous year) and in their relationship with the GP recruited (from never having met them to a close personal relationship). Patients were interviewed first and asked about their experience of using the NHS and about their relationships with GPs and practice nurses in particular. To ensure that data were gathered about particular relationships from both parties, patients were asked at the end of their interview if they would consent to their GP being interviewed about their care, with a promise that everything said in the patient interview would remain confidential. All but one patient consented.

Interviews were conducted at a convenient location for participants (usually the patient's home or the general practitioner's surgery) in 1999–2001.[2] Interviews lasted between 45 and 75 minutes, and were audiotaped (with one recording failure), transcribed, and anonymized. Initial topic guides were developed based on the literature, modified during the initial phase, and evolved throughout the study according to early analysis. All data were analyzed, including the initial phase interviews (16 interviews with GPs, 32 with patients). The focus of the analysis was on how different aspects of 'continuity' were talked about as personal continuity is claimed as a 'core value' of U.K. general practice (Guthrie and Wyke 2006). Early in data collection, it became clear that 'trust' and 'confidence' were used by both patients and GPs to explain why particular relationships were important or to justify choices made. The topic guide was therefore amended to include specific probes relating to trust. However, trust was not the primary focus of interviews, and the analysis presented here should therefore be considered preliminary, although it has been possible to identify areas for more focused research in the future.

Data management and analysis was facilitated using NVivo software as an indexing and coding tool. Validity was ensured by repeated reading of whole transcripts to keep the analysis comprehensive; by the use of a form of constant comparison using an active search for counterexamples to emerging analysis; and by modification of the topic guide in response to early analysis. Reliability was ensured through regular meetings between the main analyst and two other researchers to discuss all analytical notes written, shared analysis of a sample of transcripts, and disagreements being resolved by discussion and re-analysis (Seale 1999; Silverman 1993). No new themes emerged during analysis of interviews with GPs and patients in the final two practices, at which point it was considered that saturation had been achieved.

7.3 RESULTS

7.3.1 The Trustworthiness of Doctors

When making appointments, patients balanced preferences for *whom* to see with preferences for *when* to be seen, depending on the problem to be discussed (Guthrie and Wyke 2006). All but one of those with chronic illness had a preference for a particular doctor for nonurgent problems, whereas most of those without chronic illness prioritized when to be seen under all circumstances. When discussing urgent care, patients expressed a social trust in all doctors. Although one patient preferred to see a particular GP for his more chronic problems, in more urgent situations, any GP would do, as the following illustrates:

> "If I have to be seen quickly, I'll put that to one side obviously, you can't just say "Well I demand to see Dr. X." I mean, we're thinking about the Dr. Finlay days when the Doctor would grab his black bag and rush out to Mrs. So-and-so, because she was having a fit of the vapours or something, oh no, no, forget that. No you would put that to one side and say if it's something serious, "What I need is a qualified medical practitioner to have a look at this right now, I don't care who it is."

Social trust in doctors was justified in terms of GPs having 'been through the training' and being properly qualified, with an assumption that regulation by 'the authorities' ensured technical competence. Only one patient, a woman with long-standing alcohol problems, explicitly expressed initial distrust of doctors. Although having a doctor she trusted was important to her, her starting position with doctors she did not know was one of distrust, which could be modified in a developing relationship:

> "You've got to trust your doctor. If you don't trust your doctor, you're not going to be honest with them, and then something is going to go

wrong with you. . . . I don't trust all doctors, no. Just the ones that I get to know. You know that I can sit and talk to one to one."

Patients who actively tried to see a particular doctor did so in part because they had greater 'trust' or 'confidence' in them based on experience of care in the past. Although a few patients cited how their doctor had handled a particular major illness, such as a heart attack, for most it was repeated experience of caring, compassion, and commitment that underpinned trust:

> "Well, there's a link comes and you've got a confidence because they have cared about you and sorted things out. You get a confidence . . . I was very sick with the third child with kidney problems. He used to say to me, 'Now don't worry, I'll be there' and I always thought he would be there . . . It was just that took me through the months, you know, knowing that he'd be there and looking after me."

Although other GPs were assumed to be technically competent, the individually trusted doctor was expected to care about the patient as a person, now and in the future. Reflecting on why she tried to see *her* doctor wherever possible, one patient said:

> "I think when you're seeing different doctors, I honestly feel they're only there to help you out as far as they can that day, because you're only seeing them that day."

Interpersonal trust was therefore primarily based on judgments about the GPs' caring and compassion. Patients routinely commented on different GPs they had seen in these terms, saying they preferred *their* doctor because he or she had these characteristics:

> "He's very good, very patient, he's interested in the boy with the allergies [her son, whose illnesses are the main reason she consults]. He does show an interest. He always, even if I go with something else, he will ask about him and how I'm getting on. He's genuinely interested, and he's always got time."

In contrast, explicit judgments about technical competence were generally avoided or qualified by saying how difficult it was for the patient to know (the exception being a nurse discussing a misdiagnosis of shingles—see below). This was despite many patients saying that 'the top priority is someone who knows what they are doing and gets it right.'

Three patients said they had experienced a clear error by a doctor. For one (a nurse without chronic ill-health), a misdiagnosis of shingles made her wary of the technical competence of the doctor involved, although her preference for rapid access meant that she would still see her if necessary.

For the other two, the error was assumed to be an honest mistake by a caring person and did not alter their preference for, or future expectations of, that doctor.

Judgments about the technical competence of particular doctors were therefore either implicit or based on judgments about the doctor's motivation, interest, or the extent to which they were perceived to care. In contrast, many patients described doctors they had seen whom they had judged rude or uncaring (although several commented that they might still be medically knowledgeable). The strategy adopted in response was one of avoidance by seeking appointments with other doctors—rather than complaint or confrontation because this was perceived to risk future care. Having described a situation where she was unhappy with a doctor's manner, one patient reported that there was little value in complaining, because then you might not get the treatment that you needed.

All but one of the patients therefore described an initially blind social trust in doctors being technically competent and committed to act in their interest, justifying the validity of this by referring to (unspecified) regulators of training and practice. Over time, blind trust in particular doctors could become more grounded in judgments of interpersonal skills and the doctor's commitment to care and to act in the patient's interests and could develop a strong affective element. However, trust in technical competence remained relatively blind, as it was rarely directly judged.

GPs took it for granted that patients trusted them, based on observing that many patients chose to repeatedly consult with them (although a few acknowledged that they would not know about patients who chose to see another doctor). This was perceived as largely independent of wider changes in health care, which, as one GP remarked, did not 'change the core feeling of trust that the patients have in me,' because this interpersonal trust was assumed to grow from the development of personal relationships over time. Talking about a patient she had seen that morning, this GP initially described the consultation in terms of the problem dealt with (diarrhoea in a toddler), framing the management of the child in terms of the trusting relationship that the GP assumed existed with the mother:

> "I think it's much easier when you know the mum because I think she's known me for quite a long time and I think she trusts my [judgment], in that I've dealt with other things before and so when she came in she was quite happy when I examined the child. I think when I reassured her she was happy."

When talking about particular patients, GPs generally used the same framing of particular patients trusting them as individuals. However, several GPs were careful to qualify such statements by emphasizing that this did not reflect on the technical competence of their colleagues:

"That's an important thing to emphasize, that we're all equally good as doctors. If you were acutely ill you would be happy to see any doctor, but it's important for each of us as doctors to respect each other. If somebody is in the process of doing something with a patient you should hold back and not get involved with that process."

GPs therefore assumed that social trust existed in the sense of patients being able to trust all doctors to be technically competent and acting in good faith, although deeper interpersonal trust could develop as part of a longer relationship.

7.3.2 The Legitimacy of Patients

When talking abstractly about general practice, GPs emphasized that they were open to any kind of patient or problem, even if it was "not strictly medical." However, when asked about individual patients, GPs routinely commented on the appropriateness of their use of general practice, indicating that this openness was qualified in practice. When talking about their work in general terms, ideas of 'good' patients were frequently discussed, where the 'good' patient was one who consulted only when necessary with a problem that the doctor could have an impact on and accepted the doctor's opinion and advice.

"I would say a patient who is easy to deal with might be classed as a good patient. Somebody who possibly presents things that are not trivial, things that you can possibly answer or have some interest in, but also takes some account of your explanation and, perhaps gives you credit for knowing a bit, as in doesn't take it all on themselves to say 'this is what I need,' etc., but actually takes part in the decision-making process. And also somebody who will take their medication or will attend a hospital appointment."

When talking about particular patients the GP did not know well, this judgment was based on a quick scan of the written medical record during the interview, supplemented with some personal knowledge where available:

"She's a fairly capable, sensible sort of person who deals in a sensible manner with her children. . . . I mean that she's not the sort of person who brings her children on a regular basis for umpteen minor illnesses."

GPs made more complex or nuanced judgments when they knew patients well (usually when the patient identified them as *their* doctor). In this circumstance, personal knowledge of the patient sometimes explained or justified 'inappropriate' consultation or behaviour. Talking about one patient, whose physical illnesses were less important to him than his concerns about his disabled wife, his GP said:

> "I might think he's a fussy old git, with a troublesome wife at home. I would not like to think I thought that, but I could think that. Because you would read him, maybe, as just being an emotional, fussy man. But you see him from a totally different angle when you see the way he handles his wife, he picks her up like Dresden China, there's an emotion there, that you can therefore see where he's coming from, you understand therefore, all the other things that go on in his life."

Other patients who disagreed with doctors' diagnosis of their problem, or did not follow medical advice for treatment, were often described as 'difficult' by GPs. Again though, such behaviour could be understood and become easier to tolerate with personal knowledge.

> "She's somebody the previous GP—there were lots of references and notes about not complying with treatment . . . I think now that I've realized, whatever I do, she's not going to take advice, then I really have to deal with her symptoms as they occur. . . . Earlier on I used to sometimes be irritated by her . . . whereas now I've become slightly more tolerant to her, or accepting of her, or understanding."

However, GPs did not appear particularly vulnerable when making these judgments, with little sense of the betrayal expected in trusting relationships except under unusual circumstances:

> "The only patient that I have ever put off my list was somebody who was lying, deceitful, deliberately giving wrong telephone numbers, was deceiving a lot of other people apart from us, and quite demanding in terms of calling and demanding to be seen at home all the time in spite of us saying that clinically she didn't need to be . . . You are frustrated because you don't feel that you can do anything. And you feel you have been manipulated."

GPs' initial stance towards patients they did not know was therefore considerably more sceptical than patients' initial stance towards GPs. Within the interview, patients were routinely judged in terms of the appropriateness of their use of services or response to medical advice. These judgments became more nuanced when GPs knew the patient better, with GPs becoming more accepting of patient individuality within longer-term relationships. However, there was little sense that GPs were particularly vulnerable to feelings of betrayal except under unusual circumstances.

When talking about their use of general practice, patients frequently emphasized that they rarely attended, or only did so when it's absolutely necessary—I don't trouble them. Patients took it for granted that GPs judged the appropriateness of their use of health care, and many described situations where they felt negatively judged.

> "Sometimes I've left the doctor's surgery thinking, "Oh, God, I shouldnae have been here." It's sort of been, "You've just got one of these flu type things and you're just going to have to let it run through your system and you shouldn't have needed me to tell you 'that' feeling."

An important reason for seeing a particular doctor was that it was less necessary to justify each appointment, because *their* doctor knew that they only attended when necessary. One patient said she saw one particular GP ("my doctor") whenever possible. When asked why she preferred to see this doctor, she said:

> "I feel my doctor knows me very well and she knows the kind of person I am, that I'm not a time-waster . . . She knows that I don't moan about my health to her because I only go when it's something really that I can't deal with myself. . . . But if it's a doctor I don't know, I sit down at his desk and just wait for him to speak to me. But I have known some up there that maybe just sit (leans back in chair and crosses arms and stares at me silently). And waiting. Waiting for you to, sort of you know, "Well?" Kind of, "What are you here for?" They're not saying that but their manner is saying that."

For this patient and others, *their* doctor was assumed to trust them to use health services appropriately, which meant that they could avoid having to constantly reconstruct their legitimacy as service users. The second way in which patients perceived themselves judged was when they disagreed with diagnoses or treatment plans:

> "Well I am aware that if you start causing trouble in GPs, you get a reputation . . . Not that I'm particularly worried that my doctor would sort of strike me off or anything. But I just think it wouldn't help our relationship if I were to say, 'Well actually I think you're wrong.'"

This reticence particularly applied when seeing doctors with whom they did not have a relationship. An example is a patient who strongly preferred seeing "my GP" because he felt able to be more active in the consultation by asking questions and being involved in decision making (the GP described him as someone who "asked a lot of questions, which was a bit of a nuisance.") However, when asked how he responded when he thought GPs had made a mistake, he referred to a consultation where a GP he did not know had not measured his blood pressure as he had been expecting:

"I would go away sheepishly and not say a damned thing. As I did . . .
If someone sold you four apples, or if I asked for four apples and they
gave you two I would tend to say something. I was sitting there thinking you should be taking my blood pressure and she [a GP he doesn't
know] doesn't. I'm not inclined to do that with a doctor. You know, I'm
a wee bit wary of them . . . your life in their hands, you tend not to be
as honest as you would with say someone who is selling you a pound
of mince."

Being actively involved in the consultation by asking questions and sharing
decisions therefore appeared a potentially risky activity for patients, in that
GPs might judge their behaviour inappropriate and label them a difficult or
troublesome patient, with potential adverse consequences on future care.
Establishing a relationship with a particular GP was one way to mitigate
that risk, as patients assumed that their legitimacy was accepted by *their*
GP. However, it is important to recognise that although GPs might become
more tolerant of patients being more active when they knew them, they
still sometimes talked about this in somewhat negative ways. Describing
a patient who particularly valued seeing him because he could freely ask
questions, this GP said:

"He likes to know an awful lot and be in control a lot. You kind of
have to work around him a little bit. He always wants to know just a
little bit more about digoxin, you know—'It slows the heart does it
doctor?' And 'how does it slow the heart?' And he might come up with
his theory and it's just an interesting challenge at times with him."

Unlike GPs, patients did not take their trustworthiness or legitimacy for
granted. Rather, legitimacy was something that required repeated maintenance. Seeing *their* doctor was one way of avoiding repeated reconstruc-
tion of legitimacy with new doctors. Being accepted as legitimate in turn
was perceived to make it easier to be actively involved in consultations and
decision making.

7.4   TRUSTWORTHINESS AND ASYMMETRY
IN THE DOCTOR–PATIENT RELATIONSHIP

All but one of the patients expressed strong social trust in doctors. Where
reasons for this were given, patients referred to (vague) assumptions about
medical training and the regulation of practising doctors. The 'leap of
faith' (Möllering 2001) being made was broad, in that the expectations
formed were that any doctor would be technically competent, caring
(have empathy and interpersonal skills), and would act in the patient's
best interests (be a faithful agent). With experience of particular doctors,

then, two different kinds of leaps of faith were apparent. The first occurs when patients tried to see GPs (often one GP) of whom they had positive expectations to care and to act in their best interests. This kind of trust still required a leap of faith, but it was one with some explicit basis in personal experience and judgment of past treatment by particular individuals. On the face of it, this study therefore supports Hall's contention that 'as experience develops, the basis for trust likely shifts rapidly from system features to knowledge of individual characteristics gained from firsthand experience.' (Hall et al. 2001, 620).

In contrast, however, technical competence remained either implicit (the GP as doctor was assumed to be competent) or was inferred from judgments about interpersonal skills (the caring GP was assumed to be competent). Even when GPs were disliked because of their manner, patients often still assumed that they were technically competent and might still choose to see them when rapid access was desired (although this is at least in part, a pragmatic response to an inflexible system of access). The second leap of faith—that relating to technical competence—is therefore largely unchanged by experience and remains largely reliant on blind, social trust.

One likely reason for this difference is that patients' sense of legitimacy was relatively fragile and required constant maintenance. Patients minimized the risk of being judged illegitimate by being more cautious or passive with doctors they did not know (for example by asking fewer questions) and by avoiding doctors they mistrusted (rather than openly responding to problematic behaviour by a doctor). GPs' view of their own trustworthiness is therefore probably partly based on a misleading absence of explicit challenge. In contrast, patients' legitimacy required constant maintenance to sustain GP's perceptions of their trustworthiness. In the interviews, GPs routinely judged patients' legitimacy, and patients routinely presented themselves as *appropriate* users of health services, paralleling their descriptions of how they acted in everyday life and how they believed professionals perceived them.

> 'They now realize that I don't make appointments for the sake of appointments. I'm not wasting the doctor's time.'

Both GPs and patients therefore appeared to initially frame consultations with someone unknown in terms of a stereotype of the other person. Both are 'blind,' but patients accorded GPs intrinsic legitimacy as doctors, whereas GPs took a more sceptical stance on the legitimacy of patients. As GPs and patients got to know each other, then, judgments on both sides were informed by personal knowledge. However, asymmetry remained because patients' trust in technical competence remained blind, and because GPs' judgments about patient legitimacy were more explicit to patients than patients' judgments about GPs (un)trustworthiness were to GPs.

An explanation for this asymmetry is that trust in GP–patient relationships is framed by the wider assumption of doctors as naturally *expert* and patients as not. Expertise in the application of relatively abstract technical knowledge is the basis of all professional claims to jurisdiction over an area of work (Abbott 1988). To be a doctor is to have expertise in the diagnosis and treatment of illness and disease. Notably, it is this expert knowledge that is most privileged in this study, in the way that patients avoided making strong judgments about technical competence and in the way that patients are at risk of negative judgment when questioning or not following medical advice. In contrast, GPs' interpersonal skills relating to communication and motivation appeared more open to patient judgment and underpinned the leap of faith made to trust particular doctors. The appropriateness of patients' use of health care was also routinely judged in terms of whether patients consulted unnecessarily. This created an interesting double-bind: Knowing if a consultation was appropriate required medical knowledge that patients were assumed not to have. Talking about deciding whether to make an urgent appointment, this man said:

> Patient: "There is this question. 'Is it an emergency?' And that's when your conscience kicks in, you know, you have maybe got a searing headache. 'Is it an emergency'? Well you don't know. I mean it could be a brain tumour, it could just be a headache, it could be a migraine. Are you supposed to suffer all day and the next day before you go?"
>
> Interviewer: "So it pushes the judgment onto you?"
>
> Patient: "Well that's right, yes. If you can make the judgment. You know, nobody reasonably can unless they are seen by a doctor."

How trust is framed, and what kinds of trust are necessary, are therefore bound up with medical expertise. This expertise is itself the source of medical power, as knowledge and its application are central to professionals' claims to jurisdiction over work and to their autonomy in defining problems and their solutions (Abbott 1988).

7.5   DISCUSSION

The degree of asymmetry found in this study supports the belief that doctors lack the vulnerability identified as a necessary condition for trust and therefore calls into question whether doctors trusting patients is a meaningful concept (Hall et al. 2001). However, this assumes that such asymmetry is a natural feature of doctor–patient relationships, which is dubious given recent changes that increasingly open expert technical knowledge to lay judgment. Such judgments are seen as threats to professional autonomy and power (Harrison and Ahmad 2000; Haug 1988). These changes can be categorized in two ways.

The first relates to relationships between the state and medicine, where recognition of deficiencies in quality and safety in current medical practice (Institute of Medicine 1999, 2001) has driven growing external measurement and regulation of professional work (Harrison and Ahmad 2000), often triggered by particular failures of self-regulation (e.g., Shipman Inquiry 2004). The main effect of greater external regulation on trust is likely to be on social trust, although it may have more immediate impact in other ways, as it also acts to change relative authority over health care between the 'countervailing powers' of the state and organized medicine (Light 1993).

The second kind of change has potentially more immediate impact on individual patients. It includes technological change, such as the increasing dissemination of medical knowledge via the Internet, and the increasing policy emphasis on shared decision making, self-management of disease, and 'expert' patients, all of which emphasize respect for patient autonomy and improved quality of life (Department of Health 2006). Such changes also potentially serve purposes other than patient autonomy, such as cost containment and reducing professional power in relation to managers and the state. This emphasizes that there are multiple, legitimate interests at stake (Light 1993) that are not automatically aligned (Rosen and Dewar 2004). Balancing the social good with individual autonomy is not straight-forward, as U.K. debates over the mumps, measles, and rubella triple vaccine (Brownlie and Howson 2005, 2006) and paying for expensive drugs show (Barrett et al. 2006).

The way that these macrolevel changes play out in the care of individual patients will therefore be complex. Policies that promote the patient as expert (Dept. of Health 2006, Tuckett 1985) tend not to engage with the problems that individual patients may face in getting their particular expertise acknowledged, not least because questioning and asking to share in decisions may threaten an individual patient's legitimacy and potentially jeopardize their future care. Personal continuity, or ongoing relationships, may mitigate such risks, although current policy prioritizes rapid access to primary care over choice of which doctor to see (Guthrie and Wyke 2006).

How these considerable macrolevel changes may play out in changing social and interpersonal trust is a matter for empirical research, but it may be more helpful to consider what kind of relationship might create the conditions where doctors need to trust patients and whether such relationships are preferable. As Entwistle and Quick (2006) propose, in the context of patient safety:

> 'It may be appropriate to encourage [health professionals] to think not in terms of a loss of trust, but rather a shift in the nature of

the patient–professional relationship in which trust might occur. If patients' trust is seen less in the context of a dependency relationship and more in the context of a partnership relationship (in what is mutually acknowledged to be a somewhat risky enterprise), patients' potential contribution to their safety can be regarded as compatible with, rather than indicative of a lack of, trust.' (409)

However, in this context, patients' trust in doctors is probably less important than the implications of doctors' trusting patients. Training patients to be expert (Dept. of Health 2006), training doctors to share decision making (Elwyn et al. 2004), and other changes may make doctor–patient relationships more equal, but learning to trust patients to play a major part in technical decisions will be a painful process for many doctors, because it requires them to cede at least some professional expertise and, as result, leaves them more vulnerable. For this reason, such changes are likely to be resisted by many doctors and other health care professionals (Abbott 1988; O'Flynn and Britten 2006).

Nonetheless, Rogers (2002) makes a compelling argument that 'trust [in patients] is crucial to the development of morally respectful relationships, which in turn are central to medical practice' (80). If doctors are serious about the centrality of mutual doctor–patient relationships and respect for patient autonomy to their ethos and practice, then we need to make the leap of faith to believe that sharing knowledge with patients and involving them in decisions will mean that medical expertise will be changed rather than destroyed.

Starting from the premise that trust exists in health relationships, and that the kind of trust that is possible (or required) will depend on the nature of those relationships, there are many opportunities for future research. First, medical trust research has paid too little attention to the nature of the relationships within which trust is embedded. It takes (at least) two to make a relationship, and 'trust in doctors' ignores other ways in which both sides of a relationship are connected. As indicated above, current policy is training a cohort of patients to be more 'expert' (DOH 2006), providing an interesting opportunity to study how the deployment of this expertise changes relationships with health care professionals and impacts on trust and legitimacy within those relationships. Second, like this study, most trust research has been cross-sectional and therefore examines change only in retrospect. Longitudinal research will lead to a better understanding of how trust evolves over time, and how changing patient circumstance and developing relationships with doctors influence this. Third, this study has largely involved people of white European origin with common physical conditions where medical expertise is relatively unchallenged (diabetes, high blood pressure, ordinary acute illnesses). Other areas of medical knowledge and practice are much more contested (Barrett et al. 2006; Brownlie and Howson 2006), and experience of social and interpersonal trust may be very different for people with stigmatizing conditions (such as mental illness), or from more marginal social groups (such as minority ethnic communities or drug users). Of particular interest would be how variations in patients' assumed legitimacy influence doctors' assumed trustworthiness and how these then play out in the development of interpersonal trust within particular relationships. Finally, this study has focused on trust within individual relationships and taken social trust largely for granted. Substantial regulatory reform has been implemented, or is planned, and the impact of this on trust relations between professions, managers and the state deserves further study, both because of potential consequences on professional behaviour (O'Neill 2002) and because of the way that these frame social trust in individual professional–patient relationships.

NOTES

1. General practitioners are the sole providers of primary medical care in the U.K. and are the equivalent of U.S. family practitioners in that they care for patients unrestricted by age, gender, or condition.
2. Many of the themes highlighted in this research continue to have resonance five years later, but since the research was carried out in 2001, there have been significant changes in GP contracts in the U.K.

REFERENCES

Abbott, A. 1988. *The System of Professions*. London: Chicago University Press.

ABIM Foundation, ACP-ASIM Foundation, and European Foundation of Internal Medicine. 2002. Medical professionalism in the new millennium: A physician charter. *Annals of Internal Medicine* 136 (3): 243–246.

Ahern, M. M., and M. S. Hendryx. 2003. Social capital and trust in providers. *Social Science and Medicine* 57 (7): 1195–1203.

Barrett, A., T. Roques, M. Small, and R. D. Smith. 2006. How much will Herceptin really cost? *British Medical Journal* 333: 1118–1120.

Brownlie, J., and A. Howson. 2005. 'Leaps of faith' and MMR: An empirical study. *Sociology* 39 (2): 221–239.

———. 2006. Between the demands of truth and government: Health practitioners, trust and immunisation work. *Social Science and Medicine* 62 (2): 433–443.

Burkitt-Wright, E., C. Holcombe, and P. Salmon. 2004. Doctors' communication of trust, care, and respect in breast cancer: Qualitative study. *British Medical Journal* 328: 864–869.

Calnan, M., and E. Sanford. 2004. Public trust in healthcare: The system or the doctor? *Quality and Safety in Healthcare* 13 (2): 92–97.

Chew-Graham, C. A., C. R. May, and M. S. Perry. 2002. Qualitative research and the problem of judgement: Lessons from interviewing fellow professionals. *Family Practice* 19 (3): 285–289.

Davies, H. T. O. 1999. Falling public trust in health services: Implications for accountability. *Journal of Health Services Research and Policy* 4 (4): 193–194.

Dibben, M. R., and H. T. O. Davies. 2004. Trustworthy doctors in confidence building systems. *Quality and Safety in Healthcare* 13 (2): 88–89.

Department of Health. 2006. *The Expert Patients Programme*. London, Department of Health.

Elwyn, G., A. Edwards, K. Hood, M. Robling, C. Atwell, I. Russell, M. Wensing, and R. Grol. 2004. Achieving involvement: Process outcomes from a cluster randomised trial of shared decision making skill development and use of risk communication aids in general practice. *Family Practice* 21 (4): 337–346.

Entwistle, V. A., and O. Quick. 2006. Trust in the context of patient safety problems. *Journal of Health Organisation and Management* 20 (5): 397–416.

Fugelli, P. 2001. Trust—in general practice. *British Journal of General Practice* 51 (468): 575–579.

Gilson, L. 2006. Trust in healthcare: Theoretical perspectives and research needs. *Journal of Health Organisation and Management* 20 (5): 359–375.

Goudge, J., and L. Gilson. 2005. How can trust be investigated? Drawing lessons from past experience. *Social Science and Medicine* 61 (7): 1439–1451.

Guthrie, B., and S. Wyke. 2006. Personal continuity and access in U.K. general practice: A qualitative study of general practitioners' and patients' perceptions of when and how they matter. *BMC Family Practice* 7:11.

Hall, M. A., F. Camacho, E. Dugan, and R. Balnakrishnan. 2002. Trust in the medical professions: Conceptual and measurement issues. *Health Services Research* 37 (5): 1419–1439.

Hall, M. A., E. Dugan, B. Zheng, and A. K. Mishra. 2001. Trust in physicians and medical institutions: What is it, can it be measured, and does it matter? *The Milbank Quarterly* 79 (4): 613–639.

Hammersley, M. 1992. *What's Wrong with Ethnography: Methodological Explorations*. London: Routledge.

Harrison, S., and I. U. Ahmad. 2000. Medical autonomy and the UK state 1975 to 2025. *Sociology* 34 (1): 129–146.

Haug, M. R. 1988. A re-examination of the hypothesis of physician deprofessionalisation. *Milbank Quarterly* 66 suppl. 2: 48–56.

Institute of Medicine. 1999. *To Err is Human: Building a Safer Health System*. Washington DC: Institute of Medicine.

———. 2001. *Crossing the Quality Chasm: A New Health System for the 21st Century*. Washington DC: Institute of Medicine.

Jacobs, A. K. 2005. Rebuilding an enduring trust in medicine: A global mandate. *Circulation* 111 (25): 3494–3498.

Kao, A. C., D. C. Green, A. M. Zaslavsky, J. P. Koplan, and P. D Cleary. 1998. The relationship between method of physician payment and patient trust. *The Journal of the American Medical Association* 280 (19): 1708–1714.

Keating, N. L., D. C. Green, A. C. Kao, J. A. Gazmarian, V. Y. Wu , and P. D. Cleary. 2002. How are patients' specific ambulatory care experiences related to trust, satisfaction, and considering changing physicians? *Journal of General Internal Medicine* 17 (1): 29–39.

Light, D. W. 1993. Countervailing power: The changing character of the medical profession in the United States. In *The Changing Medical Profession: An International Perspective*. Oxford: Oxford University Press.

Mechanic, D. 1996. Changing medical organisation and the erosion of trust. *The Milbank Quarterly* 74 (2): 171–189.

Mechanic, D., and S. Meyer. 2000. Concepts of trust among patients with serious illness. *Social Science and Medicine* 51 (5): 657–668.

Möllering, G. 2001. The nature of trust: From Georg Simmel to a theory of expectation, interpretation and suspension. *Sociology* 35 (2): 403–420.

O'Flynn, N., and N. Britten. 2006. Does the achievement of medical identity limit the ability of primary care practitioners to be patient-centred? *Patient Education and Counselling* 60 (1): 49–56.

O'Neill, O. 2002. Called to account: 2002 Reith Lectures [online], [cited. . . .]. Available from <www.bbc.co.uk/radio4/reith2002/>

Pearson, S. D., and L. H. Raeke. 2000. Patients' trust in physicians: Many theories, few measures, and little data. *Journal of General Internal Medicine* 15 (7): 509–513.

Power, M. 2003. Evaluating the audit explosion. *Law and Policy* 25 (3): 185–202.

RCGP. 2004. *The Future of General Practice: A statement by the Royal College of General Practitioners*. London: RCGP.

RCGP, General Practitioners' Committee of the BMA, and NHS Alliance. 2001. *Valuing General Practice*. London: RCGP.

Rogers, W. A. 2002. Is there a moral duty for doctors to trust patients? *Journal of Medical Ethics* 28 (2): 77–80.

Rosen, R., and S. Dewar. 2004. *On Being a Doctor: Redefining Medical Professionalism for Better Patient Care*. London: Kings Fund Publications.

Seale, C. 1999. *The Quality of Qualitative Research*. London: Sage.

Secretary of State for Health. 2007. *Trust, Assurance and Safety—the Regulation of Health Professionals in the 21st Century*. Norwich: HMSO.

Shipman Inquiry Fifth Report: *Safeguarding Patients: Lessons from the Past—Proposals for the Future*. 2004. Norwich: HMSO.

Silverman, D. 1993. *Interpreting Qualitative Data*. London: Sage.

Strathern, M., ed. 2000. *Audit Cultures: Anthropological Studies in Accountability, Ethics and the Academy*. London: Routledge.

Thom, D. H., and B. Campbell. 1997. Patient–physician trust: An exploratory study. *Journal of Family Practice* 44 (2): 169–176.

Thom, D. H., M. A. Hall, and L. G. Pawlson. 2004. Measuring patient's trust in physicians when assessing quality of care. *Health Affairs* 23 (4): 124–132.

Thorne, S. E., and C. A. Robinson. 1989. Guarded alliance: Health care relationships in chronic illness. *IMAGE Journal of Nursing Scholarship* 21 (3): 153–157.

Tuckett, D. 1985. *Meetings Between Experts: An Approach to Sharing Ideas in Medical Consultations*. London: Tavistock.

Van der Schee, E., P. P. Groenewegen, and R. D. Friele. 2006. Public trust in health care: A performance indicator. *Journal of Health Organisation and Management* 20 (5): 468–476.

8 Tokens of Trust or Token Trust?
Public Consultation and 'Generation Scotland'

Gill Haddow and
Sarah Cunningham-Burley

8.1 INTRODUCTION

Large-scale genetic databases are being developed across many different countries as health-related genetics research moves to include population-level studies. Research involving large populations (with people not necessarily affected by genetic conditions and the world of the clinic) evokes a range of concerns for the different groups involved. Recognition of this has led to considerable debate about the ethical, legal and social issues in policy and research communities as well as within the wider public sphere. Such concerns find expression in a variety of ways: a renewed worry about the spectre of eugenics; recognition of the risks of unanticipated consequences; and anxiety about data security, privacy and potential breaches of trust. Such concerns are, of course, not unique to the collection and use of DNA for population-level research. However, particular issues come together in this context, making questions of trust of interest for those managing the research process, as well as for those more widely concerned with science/society relations. Research participants are asked to donate DNA for future research, with no direct benefit to themselves and no short-term health gain for the population more generally. Trust, a slippery and relational concept, is invoked in this transaction, and it is seen as necessary for the effective and acceptable development of DNA databases. However, trust's specific dimensions, in relation to genetic databases for health research, require empirical investigation, for they may not be as they seem, nor as necessary for participation and donation as assumed.

Two wider trends need to be considered, by way of setting the scene for what follows: first, the foregrounding of the 'problem of trust' in science/society relations and, second, the invocation of public understanding of, and public engagement in, science as a corrective to a perceived corrosion of trust. 'The problem of trust' has been widely critiqued and theorized in relation to human genetics (see, e.g., Jones and Salter 2003; Wynne

2006). Endemic to the condition of late modernity, scepticism and lack of trust in expert and abstract systems arise from the risks associated with technological developments. Uncertainty about risks generates mistrust and leads to demands for heightened regulation and surveillance, and with them, further dependence on abstract systems (Beck 1997; Giddens 1991). The mantra about a lack of trust or confidence in techno-science is often repeated in policy documents and in other arenas where the institutions of science confront their publics. The need to build public confidence and trust is seen as paramount, as the House of Lords Select Committee Report (2000) delineates:

> 'Society's relationship with science is in a critical phase. Science today is exciting and full of opportunities. Yet public confidence in scientific advice has been rocked by BSE and many people are uneasy about the rapid advance of areas such as biotechnology and IT even though for everyday purposes they take science and technology for granted. This crisis of confidence is of great importance both to the British Society and to British Science.'

However, such pleas for building confidence in the face of loss of public authority for science and a sense of widespread mistrust must not be taken at face value. Wynne's critique (2006) suggests the construction of a 'creation myth,' in which the problem of 'the public mistrust of science' assumes a previous era, when trust was evident and also implies that the public is a homogenous entity that holds or withholds trust. Theoretical and empirical evidence suggests a much more contextual, experiential and ambivalent picture of trust (Cunningham-Burley 2006; Khodyakov 2007; Wynne 1996).

The need for public dialogue is frequently invoked as a way to revive public trust. However, this too is part of a wider trend across policy domains of increased public involvement in debates and decision-making. In relation to science/society relations though, public engagement is envisaged as a panacea for a troubled relationship between science and the wider public and a way of building confidence in science. Thus, the same report quoted above also appeals for increased and integrated dialogue:

> 'There has been a cultural change in the attitude of most British scientists, in favour of public outreach activities. Activities to improve the public understanding of science now receive support from Government and industry. However, the crisis of trust has produced a new mood for dialogue. In addition to seeking to improve public understanding of their work, scientists are beginning to understand its impact on society and on public opinion.' (House of Lords Select Committee Report 2000 op cit).

This mood of greater transparency and dialogue has rhetorically replaced calls for increased scientific literacy amongst an 'ignorant' public as a way of promoting trust in and acceptance of scientific developments, although the 'deficit model' (which stresses public ignorance of science and identifies improved scientific literacy as important for trust and confidence in science) is still alive and well, just below the surface of the new discourse of public engagement (Irwin 2006). With increased funding for a range of work and the growing involvement of social scientists, public engagement activities and research are taking centre stage in science/society relations. This chapter draws on our experience of one such endeavor so that we can begin to reflect on issues of trust, and, following Wynne, ask whether and where there is mistrust, in what contexts and for what reasons. We shall also consider the extent to which public consultation about and engagement with genetic databases can influence the institutional constraints of science and thus scientific practice, as well as encourage reflective practice amongst all those involved in the development and use of genetic databases for health research.

After describing Generation Scotland and the associated public consultation research, we then focus on the different dimensions of trust displayed in the 'upstream' public engagement component of the developing database. Upstream refers here to public consultation and engagement at a very early stage of scientific developments, before major decisions are made and agendas set. We provide an analysis of data from focus groups with 'publics' and interviews with stakeholders. This analysis identifies different forms of trust, or lack of trust, and explores the cultural tropes and personal experiences that are used by participants to justify positions. We then consider how participants thought that issues of trust might be resolved through research governance and public engagement before offering some conclusions about the role of public engagement in shaping the context and production of a genetic database.

8.2   GENERATION SCOTLAND

The aim of Generation Scotland is to create an ethically sound family and population-based infrastructure to identify the genetic basis of common complex diseases such as cancer, stroke, heart disease and mental health problems. The concept and associated program have developed over several years and now involve three complementary projects: the Scottish Family Health Study; Genetic Health in the 21st Century; and the Donor DNA Databank. The Scottish Family Health Study will recruit a cohort of 50,000 individuals. In addition to understanding the etiology of complex diseases, Generation Scotland also aims to create more effective treatments, and it is argued that the whole program and its associated infrastructure will be to the overall medical, social and economic benefit of Scotland and its people. Generation Scotland is very much a partnership, involving the Scottish University Medical Schools, Biomedical Research Institutes, the National Health Service in Scotland and, of course, the people of Scotland. It currently receives funding from the Scottish Executive Chief Scientist's Office and the Scottish Higher Education Funding Council. Its website (www.generationscotland.org) highlights the importance of the relationship between the public and the project with the following statement:

> 'A principle aim of Generation Scotland it to keep participants and the wider public informed about the project and it will strive to build a relationship of trust. In addition Generation Scotland has embarked on a programme of public consultation. This is in order to work together in deciding the ways in which the resource is developed and used, and the benefits are shared. (www.generationscotland.org)'

8.2.1   Public Consultation and Public Engagement

Partnership between scientists, social scientists and lawyers has formed an essential part of the process and progress of Generation Scotland as it grapples with the complex ethical, legal and social issues (ELSI) that such an endeavour brings. One of the contributions of the ELSI program is concurrent consultation research with publics and stakeholders, with resultant discussions and negotiations about various aspects of the developing scientific programme, including research protocols and governance. Issues around open consent loom large, alongside data security and future use; each of these is raised by those participating in consultation activities in different fora and contexts. Thus, the Generation Scotland program, as currently configured, is actively attending to issues of public trust through public engagement, taking seriously the calls for dialogue and the putative 'crisis of trust' that spawned it.

8.3   EARLY CONSULTATION: RESEARCH METHODS

Calls for 'upstream engagement'—that is, greater public involvement at earlier stages in scientific and technological innovation—have recently been made in order to challenge current innovation processes and open them up to greater public scrutiny and involvement (Willis and Wilsdon 2004). It is argued that without early participation in the innovation process, the scope to influence the content and direction of science is foreclosed, and the focus becomes much more on downstream impacts. However, the extent to which upstream engagement can really provide an inclusive and more democratic basis for public/science relations is still an open question, as it will demand shared decision-making within new forms of dialogue. In the initial phase of Generation Scotland, early consultation was encouraged and funded; this can partly be characterized as an upstream engagement, as the project was a concept or a proposal, not a defined program of funded research. This work involved a one day public event, focus group discussions with diverse publics and interviews with specialists. The focus group discussions and interviews form the basis of our analysis here; an analysis of the public event formed part of another project (Kerr, Cunningham-Burley and Tutton 2007).

Seventeen in-depth interviews were conducted with individuals, mainly from Scotland, with varied and diverse expertise, broadly defined as 'specialists' in key fields of relevance to DNA databases (e.g., geneticists, lawyers, theologians, social scientists and clinicians) between April and July 2003. Subsequently, between January and March 2004, ten focus groups were conducted in various locations across Scotland. Groups were purposively sampled and chosen to reflect a range of demographic characteristics (gender, ethnicity and age), interests (patient, voluntary and civic groups) and localities (rural or city). The overall aim was for diversity in terms of social location rather than representation. Box 1 identifies the different groups and different specialists; the notation used throughout the rest of the chapter identifies which group or interviewee is being referred to. For the focus groups, the respondent talking is also given a reference, where possible (R1, R2 etc.).

We chose these asymmetric research methods in order to maximize discussion with the different participants. The specialists can be considered stakeholders, who would have already thought about and perhaps even contributed to discussions about Generation Scotland in particular, and certainly about genetics and health more generally. We anticipated that it would be likely that one-to-one, semistructured interviews would not be threatening and would allow detailed exploration of their points of view and ideas for creating a socially acceptable and ethically robust genetic database. On the other hand, although accepting 'lay expertize' and recognizing the diverse experience that publics bring to debates about genetics and health (Kerr, Cunningham-Burley and Amos 1998) we anticipated that detailed discussion of a proposed project in a new field of research (population genetics) might lend itself better to a focus group format rather than an individual interview. This would allow broad discussion to take place about something 'yet to happen' in an area participants may not have previously given much attention to.

In both the public and specialist components of this preliminary and exploratory consultation, we were keen to explore a range of issues. Although there was some variation both within and between the two research groups—the specialists and the publics—we used a broadly similar topic guide for both the individual interviews and the focus groups, reflecting our aim of not reinforcing an expert/lay divide. Open-ended questioning during the interviews and focus groups examined issues such as participation, access, feedback, confidentiality, engagement and governance. We sought not to lead any of the discussion but to allow participants to frame the contours of the debate. We encouraged participants to raise issues themselves, to be candid about their concerns and to draw specifically on their own areas of interest and expertise as well as provide more general comment. Participants sometimes spoke from their own point of view but also commented on how they thought others might think or react.

In the focus groups, especially, a combination of the open-ended approach to discussing issues, and the preliminary stage at which we were holding them, sometimes led to respondents expressing frustration to the moderators facilitating the group. Although we had precirculated information on Generation Scotland, it was necessarily vague as the project was not clearly defined. Questions and statements such as 'What are the options?' (FG1 R3), and 'I don't know, I don't know enough yet' (FG1 R2) illustrate this occasional frustration and demonstrate the challenge of doing research at this stage and on a complex issue. Some of this dissatisfaction was also present in the one-to-one interviews, although to a lesser extent, as the broad contours of research design and potential governance arrangements were more familiar territory. However, across the board, we also found participants to be keen to talk and pleased to be involved in discussions about Generation Scotland.

All groups had a moderator to conduct the discussion and a rapporteur for capturing the salient points and interjecting probes as appropriate. Most discussions and all interviews were also audiorecorded and transcribed. The analysis of the corpus began inductively, with the transcripts and accompanying notes being read closely by the researchers and then sorted into themes. We then gave these chunks of text labels such as 'access' or 'participation' before returning to each for further analytical detail and searching for relationships; trust was a cross-cutting theme. Hence, a combination of a thematic content analysis and a constant comparative method were used. All identifying information has been removed from the following accounts; quotes are used illustratively to reinforce the analytical points and the attribution clarifies the focus group or interview from which it was drawn.

There are differences between the interview and focus group accounts in terms of issues raised and depth of discussion, but there was also a considerable degree of commonality and overlap, for example about factors that would affect participation and trust. We explore accounts of what trust means to people, trying to consider issues of interpretation and context (Möllering 2001). We draw upon extracts where the participants make explicit and spontaneous reference to trust. We outline reasons for trusting or not trusting one organization or 'expert' over another and the reasons for 'leaps of faith' (Brownlie and Howson 2005), 'suspension' (Möllering 2001) or 'as if' trust (Lewis and Weigert 1985; Giddens 1991; Wynne 1996).

8.4   EXPLORING TRUST

8.4.1   Trust in Scientific Progress

By and large, the initial reaction to Generation Scotland was positive from most focus group participants and specialist interviewees, with a strong endorsement of the future benefits to society. Focus-group participants viewed Generation Scotland as a good use of resources because of the attention on the 'big three' diseases (cancer, heart disease and mental health); these common diseases seemed to resonate with people's own concerns and experiences. The wider public and specialists also identified other diseases that might be appropriate to investigate, such as multiple sclerosis—a disease that has high prevalence in Scotland—other degenerative diseases and asthma. The rationale for Generation Scotland was thus endorsed, suggesting an overall trust in scientific progress and the genetic approach to understanding and treating disease. So, rather than evoking mistrust, this large, family-based population genetic database fitted into normative expectations about the role of medical science in moderating disease and promoting health. The cognitive authority of genetic science was mostly sustained rather than challenged in focus groups and interviews, as the following extract from a focus group discussion suggests:

> **Respondent 1:** Personally, I think it's long overdue. I'm really pleased that you're talking about building a Scottish picture. And you're drawing together a lot of information on treatments and service and so on that needs to be done because I think we need to identify where the system falls down, where it works. You're not going to get overnight results or benefits from it, but somebody has to take the first step and start pulling all this together. It may not be this generation, even the next that gets the full benefits. I've got two wee granddaughters and I'd like to think that by the time they were adults that the service was a lot more clear-cut and efficient and targeted. I'll get off my soapbox now.

> **Respondent 2:** You've got to really look longer-term. It's all very well everybody that's affected or family that's affected or that, they'll be saying that money could help them now. But if nobody does it for the future we'll just never get off the bit. (FG4).

The idea of future benefit, as yet unknown, might have been thought to evoke uncertainty and concern, or at least ambivalence, yet this does not seem to be the case. However, as we go on to explore, issues relating to future uses was one area where trust might be undermined.

A sense of trust was evoked in a range of comments about professional ethics and practice. One participant noted that health professionals 'take an oath not to disclose your business' (FG10). Any unauthorized divulgence of information would be liable for prosecution, which some found reassuring. Some participants were unsure whether they trusted scientists, but comments such as 'if they are clever enough to be doing this, they should be trusted because who else will be able to help' (FG6) suggest a relationship between trust and knowledge that was repeated in other groups. As participants in Focus Group 10 noted, without having 'faith,' presumably in scientific progress and the actions of medical scientists and clinicians, diseases like dementia would never be eradicated and 'nothing comes without some risk' (FG10). This suggests that trust and awareness of risk can go hand-in-hand. The following discussion about trust, expertise and knowledge occurred in the Seniors' (older people's) group:

Respondent 2: I would think anything that's, at the end of the day going to be good for the people would probably be worth trying. I would have no objection.

Interviewer: So something like this project, you think it might have benefits for the people of Scotland? Or?

Respondent 2: I imagine people in [indecipherable] so we need to trust them.

Interviewer: Would you trust them?

Respondent 2: I think so.

Interviewer: Where does that trust come from? Because they're medical geneticists and . . .

Respondent 2: They have the knowledge, I hope, they have been researching and have obviously medical knowledge that I don't have. So from that point of view I would trust them.

Interviewer: So the idea in itself, from your point of view, seems like a good one?

Respondent 2: Yes. (FG2).

'At the end of the day' is an interesting term used in everyday discussions and suggests a consequentialist view that, despite risks in following a particular course of action, the outcome is the most important element. In this exchange about trust, therefore, because medical geneticists are thought to have the specific knowledge to bring about the anticipated benefits, this single goal should evoke trust, albeit rather conditionally expressed.

8.4.2 Homegrown Trust

A further feature of the trust that seemed to be placed in Generation Scotland, hinted at in the quote above from Focus Group 4, was its particular Scottish focus. This Scottish dimension was also stressed by several of the specialist interviewees, and Scottish ownership of Generation Scotland was understood as a positive element in a number of ways, including, as the following clinical geneticist suggested, evoking trust and encouraging participation:

> 'I suspect the public can see it as being owned within Scotland, by Scottish academia and Scottish health, can see the involvement of individuals locally that they are aware of and therefore in general trust, because they've used them or their relatives have used them (. . . .) I think Generation Scotland would have, as its name implies, a greater impact locally because it is a locally driven thing. I think that's quite important.' (Clinical Geneticist).

A combination of local experience and national pride seems to be evoked here, and the respondent thinks this will inform public attitudes. Unlike the distance and suspicion towards unknown others, which we explore below, here is a suggestion that the basis of trust—experiential knowledge and previous social relationships—is embedded in locale and local relationships.

Previous experience seemed to be important, and several stories were recounted in focus groups of research-based clinical encounters. The example below demonstrates the positive nature of this, reinforcing the perception of medical science in a clinical context as a worthwhile and trustworthy endeavor with sometimes unanticipated health benefits:

> **Respondent 3:** I think on the other hand, speaking for myself, my GP asked me to take part in a little research project up at the hospital. When I went up there, thinking it was just an hour's test and then I'd get away, they actually traced something that needed treated and said 'you need this right away.' I was very glad to have that information. I was quite happy beforehand, I knew nothing about it, but I was happy that they told me. . . . (FG2).

8.4.3 Willingness to Participate as a Token of Trust

Although the factors influencing participation are varied and extend beyond a signal of trust, participation and donation of DNA can be conceptualized as a token of trust, and the focus-group discussions suggested that social location was relevant. Patient or support groups were more likely to express a willingness to participate, suggesting again that relational aspects of trust are important, in the context of personal experience of disease and medical intervention

(Haddow, Laurie, Cunningham-Burley and Hunter 2007). However, trust in future benefits, as described above, was also implicit in the reasons given for likely participation: a few seemed to express a kind of moral obligation to take part for the sake of their children or grandchildren.

Specialists tended to talk about the likely participation of others (the wider public) rather than whether they themselves would participate. Reflecting the focus group analyses, they proposed that those directly affected by disease would be more likely to participate and those more distant, emotionally or geographically, less likely:

> 'I would have thought if anything a family-linked one is more likely to get participation and support because it's more obvious that one, if you were marketing this you can say that immediate benefits of the need of doing this are more obvious to families that have been affected by a serious medical condition that might have some genetic underpinning. Whereas why on earth would a bunch of otherwise apparently healthy people pitch up to give blood and have their genes examined and stored?' (Public Health Specialist).

8.5 EXPLORING LACK OF TRUST

8.5.1 Breaching Trust

Although an overall sense of optimism suffused accounts from the interviews and focus groups, this was tempered by concerns and sometimes overt expressions of scepticism and mistrust. Generalized and specific instances of breaches of trust are culturally available and were drawn upon by participants, modifying their positive reactions to Generation Scotland and demonstrating their awareness of distant processes over which they have little control. The following exchange was from the focus group in a rural area:

> Respondent 1: That's it, they're doing what they say they're going to be doing that the samples you would give would be used for the reasons, only for the purposes of these illnesses, these diseases, these ailments, solely for that purpose. And I think people are sceptical about whether that will probably happen. You hear from the news every day for whatever area of work or business or NHS or whatever, you hear of just organizations breaching trust, breaching confidentiality, we hear it every day.

> Respondent 5: Even our own lives.

> Respondent 3: And it's sad.

Respondent 1: And so I think that makes people very sceptical to actually trust what a big organization is saying to you. You've been promised to only use your blood sample for this, this and this. Probably wouldn't [indecipherable] because I think we've all heard, and we've been fed so many untruths about how people were deceived and were used in the past . . .

Respondent 4: But we donate our blood, we give blood.

Respondent 1: But you only, you give your blood on a specific . . . you're giving it for specific reasons. The reasons that when you're giving blood are written down and you're trusting that they're using your blood for what you agreed to when you signed for. (FG5).

Aspects of language-use suggest a distrust of abstract institutions and unknown others—references to 'they' or 'big organization.' However, even in this exchange a counterargument is presented of a trustworthy organization, the Scottish National Blood Transfusion Service, which receives and manages donated blood. This is a locally embedded public institution, and its juxtaposition with the unknown, amorphous large organization is particularly telling; the issue of blood donation and the associated service was mentioned in a few of the focus groups.

8.5.2   Runaway Science

Although there was overall support for medical science, the focus group discussions also contained references to culturally available tropes suggestive of runaway science and the abuse of science. Cloning and eugenics are the popular references, and these may be evoked as a way of providing grounds for a generalized mistrust. An intense opposition to 'cloning' was voiced, even though this is not part of the Generation Scotland program and was not mentioned in any information provided to participants. Despite claims that cloning a person was thought unlikely it was still said to be a fear by some. For some of the older respondents, discussions about genetics brought back disturbing memories of Nazi eugenics—cloning and eugenics are both referred to in the quote below as a way of expressing concerns:

Respondent 2: I just don't like the idea of trying to copy a human being. Because I think we're all very original. I mean I'm a Christian anyway. So we're all original and that is the beauty of each individual human being and to make someone, an identical twin is the closest thing you can get to that, which is quite useful to have two but then they're not the same person are they? And this is something that I just feel so strongly about. I lived through the war and it just makes me think of

Hitler and all the terrible things he tried to do. It just horrifies me really. (FG2).

Where these issues were raised in the focus groups, cloning was a clear line that should not be crossed and a total ban was the proffered solution, in line with current legislation in the United Kingdom for reproductive cloning.

The main research area of concern, mentioned spontaneously by specialist interviewees, was behavioural genetics, where caution was advocated by a number to avoid the creation of a genetic underclass:

> 'I don't think I'm very keen on behavioural genetics, as an area of importance for the Scottish population. There's been studies done on homosexuality, there's been studies looking at some behavioural characteristics like aggression etc. and I think in general a) they're extremely iffy studies but b) I can see why understanding human diversity is a wonderful thing to do. I think in behavioural genetics one would have to be very cautious about the studies that were proposed and make sure that you ensure that they are likely to have value to the population rather than discriminate against a subgroup in some way.' (Medical Geneticist).

8.5.3   Use and Abuse of Personal Data

Generation Scotland is careful to state that all uses will be health-related and ethically approved. However, the possibility of abusing the information or data was raised, and the relationship between trust and uncertainty was discernible in discussions. For example, fears were voiced about whether an enemy might use the information in the database to develop genetic or chemical weapons:

> Who's to say that the database couldn't also be used for chemical warfare? (FG5).

These broad and abstract fears were complemented in discussions by more specific references to examples of abuse. One specialist, for example, raised the issue of rogue scientists and the impact this has on public trust, especially in the context of genetic research, which is characterized in the quote as raising particular concerns anyway:

> 'And even though I firmly believe that most researchers are doing an absolutely independent and honest job, it only takes the odd person who's falsifying the results by inventing patients in their surgery, or whatever it happens to be, to cause a great deal of ill feeling and scepticism about the entire endeavour. It's on the back of that I think that people will have concerns about Generation Scotland because it's got

everything. It's got the kind of scientific bit that people are dubious about and it's got genetics.' (Lawyer).

Other illustrations were discussed during the focus groups and interviews relating to the use/abuse of genetic data. For example, one specialist raised the issue of police access via a court order, which would be possible in exceptional circumstances. This concern was expressed using the familiar metaphor of 'big brother' and spread beyond the possibility of police use:

'The main concerns will be the sort of more George Orwellian "big brother," somebody's got samples on me. Will they be misused, literally misused in terms of forensic incrimination for example, police activity, police having access? I think at a lesser level people will be concerned with whether they may be used in terms of talking to insurance, life insurance companies or health insurance companies or in terms of medicals related to employment and things like that. There may be some sensitivities then quite specifically within family groups, when you get into the genetics of this you find that somebody's father wasn't quite who they thought their father was. A number of studies would suggest that up to 10 percent of fathers are not who the child thought the father was, so that there's sensitivity there. Those kind of things.' (Specialist in Public Health).

Although the specter of police access was not raised elsewhere, the Orwellian 'big brother' trope was also brought up in the focus groups:

Respondent 2: A lot of people might just regard this as another stage into the 'big brother' issue sort of thing . . . (FG1).

It was thought that insurance company access was inappropriate and might lead to nonparticipation. The patient-support focus groups were especially concerned that if potential employers, insurance companies or banks were able to obtain personal, medical and genetic information, it would be severely detrimental to them as individuals. Mention was made, in one patient group, of problems already experienced with insurance and gaining a mortgage. This group foresaw problems with employment, suggesting this concern was grounded in direct experience:

Respondent 1:. . . . you were talking about the companies that make the drugs, insurance companies who want to find out people's background obviously if they're trying to get insurance or different things like that, have they got leanings towards any problems later in life?

Respondent 3: That's my main worry about a database like this. Obviously (. . .) I've already had problems with insurance. I've just got a mortgage and that was a bit difficult as well. But, if you're saying that you're going to put data in the database to try and protect the people that are going to have problems . . . . obviously if you're quite healthy at the moment and you're getting insurance and different things fine, but then if they're predicted to have something is that then going to affect them say getting employment, getting a house, getting different insurance and things? That's my worst worry is learning a bit too much about people. (FG1).

These concerns ran through the focus groups with the public as well as the specialist interviews, although one academic researching genetics and insurance noted that genetic information is of little actuarial interest when calculating risk. The point rather is that the potential for access beyond medical research and its impact on individual wellbeing was raised as a concern and this can be seen as another reason for mistrust in abstract and distant processes.

8.5.4 Commercial Access for Health-Related Research

Although there was some evidence, particularly from patient-support groups, that pharmaceutical companies were perceived as a 'necessary evil' and among specialists that this was the 'way of the world,' there was also a degree of ambivalence and scepticism about commercial use of Generation Scotland data for health-related purposes (see Haddow et al 2007 for a more detailed discussion of this issue). The following example from a clinical geneticist makes reference to the specific issue of commercial involvement by the company DeCode in the Icelandic genetic database (Rose 2001), to show how commercial interests of 'an amorphous body' would jeopardize trust. The respondent talks both personally and about how others might feel:

'But what I would not like to see is the entire subsection of the study being handed to Glaxo (a pharmaceutical company) to look for genes involved in asthma. A bit the way DeCode took over Iceland, that sort of thing. I think in general, populations of both professionals and the public would be happier to think that the key to the whole thing was held by the people who started up the study and agreed to do the study, the people that they identify as being predominantly those that they would trust in their society. I think if you start handing over the whole of the study to an amorphous body that you have no control over, where they're driven by completely different aims, then I would think I'd have a problem.' (Clinical Geneticist)

The same perspectives on pharmaceutical companies were apparent in the focus groups and other specialist interviews. Different motivations, including profit, potentially jeopardize the 'public good' motive supported so willingly by respondents when thinking about Generation Scotland:

Respondent 4: I think I just wouldn't trust that there wasn't a, kind of big business (which) wouldn't have ulterior motives behind it, to cash in on this thing, so that instead of this being a very good, a positive thing. That there isn't just a kind of money-making opportunity behind it for certain people. (FG5).

Indeed, it was medical personnel, academics or research scientists that were mentioned in focus groups as those who should have access to the Generation Scotland database. It seems that trustworthy science demands trustworthy institutions and individuals.

8.5.5   Privacy

Much was made of the potential for inadvertent disclosure of kinship relationships in the focus groups. There was some concern, for example, about revealing the true nature of the kinship connections ('It would be a big blow for you to find out that the sister you think is your sister is not your sister, it's your mother' FG5). The problem of revealing information about the nature of kinship connections was viewed by a few of the specialists as inevitable in this type of genetic research (although it was also pointed out that researchers are bound by an obligation of confidentiality).

On more practical issues, there was a degree of unease around the physical storage of data about whether GP surgeries could maintain confidentiality, and there were also questions raised around the ability of the Generation Scotland organization to keep the information secure. Questions asked included: Could Generation Scotland employees steal the information? How will it be kept? And how would any conflict of interests be resolved? Can the computers be made secure enough? Discussion in the focus groups suggested that safeguards should be similar to the current level of confidentiality protecting medical records. A number of specialists suggested that there should be a requirement for legal sanctions against those who subvert confidentiality and legal protection for those who might be harmed by it. The organization of science, then, was opened up for scrutiny, and there seemed to be no assumption of trust in processes and procedures, unlike the implicit trust in the overall thrust of medical scientific progress.

Issues of privacy and confidentiality loomed quite large in the focus group discussions, as the following examples suggest:

Respondent 3: I just don't trust the government in that sense. I don't trust anyone with secrecy.

Respondent 2: It's like all the sperm donors who thought they were giving anonymously then twenty years later confronted by a son or daughter.

Interviewer: How does anybody else feel?

Respondent 1: I think he's got a point. I worked as a hospital porter many years ago during the summer, and I got access to medical records I had no business getting access to. I was told to go and collect them. How does someone feel that anyone like me just wandered in reading all your medical records? (FG3).

There are different narratives about secrecy/privacy in this discussion. The first, by R3, reflects a generalized mistrust in abstract institutions; the second, by R2, is the variability of norms of secrecy/privacy over time, with the example of challenges to anonymity with changes in regulations about sperm donation; finally R1 admits to having had unrestricted access to medical information of the highest sensitivity. Procedures to ensure privacy are thus known to be easily breached, something that the specialists too seem acutely aware of:

'I think if people have evil intent it's very difficult to stop them [accessing data] if they have enough brains. I am told that it really is virtually impossible to have unbreakable codes. And . . . [name] who is an encryption expert and he said that it's very difficult but that you can perhaps place controls on databases by controlling how they can be interrogated. Because apparently people have managed to work out in some local authority where people were looking at HIV carrier status, that it is virtually entirely the black population in some small area that are HIV carriers, and that's because they could ask questions from the database in a way that allowed them to deduce this sort of information. And then it got publicized. So one has to put controls on how the database is used, and people need to sign agreements on confidentiality and they need to be prosecuted if they break [it]. I think that's really the only thing one can do to develop sanctions against people who break the rules. But we're always going to have crooks in society I guess.' (Human Geneticist).

8.6 GENERATING TRUST IN GENERATION SCOTLAND

8.6.1 Education and the Media

The specialists made much of how the media would affect public participation and, therefore, implicitly public trust. There was recognition that expectations might not be met, and the media needs to be tempered:

'I think there is a need for considerably more education about the complexities of genetics. I think it's probably presented in a too black and white manner by much of the media and I think we need to temper that because we must not raise expectations too high. I think we have to be realistic and honest about what we might glean from such a study.' (Human Geneticist).

On the other hand, the media were a key resource in encouraging participation:

> 'I think you just manipulate the media really, just use whatever resources there are. One very obvious way of doing it I think is to convince somebody in BBC Scotland that they want to do a documentary about it. That works wonders, if you've got someone like Frontline Scotland to do a program on Generation Scotland, you'd be amazed at the publicity it would get, and the newspapers and so on.' (Specialist in Medical Law).

Here there is an implicit reliance on a deficit model of public understanding of science, where more knowledge is considered necessary to encourage participation: The serious media (documentaries) have a role to play in public education. There was also talk of public ignorance in some of the focus groups:

> '. . . Scottish people, if they don't understand something they won't just easily swallow it. They're suspicious and hold back, so you've really got a big public relations difficulty I think really in persuading people that it's a good idea, they understand it and then they go along with it.' (FG2)

8.6.2   Transparency and Feedback

A robust claim for information, and then consultation, was made in the focus groups and also for the related importance of getting Generation Scotland into the public consciousness and the popular press—'in *The Daily Record* (a local newspaper) and not the *Lancet*' (FG4). General feedback to participants was considered to be key, and individuals in the focus groups said they would be happy to participate in Generation Scotland if given regular general feedback. One respondent gave an example of not hearing anything more about clinical research at a University that he had been involved in, something he found disappointing, though he recognized that some research may take a long time to produce results (FG6).

A lack of feedback was said in the focus groups to weaken trust in Generation Scotland as the following discussion from the Edinburgh Cyclists group demonstrates:

> **Respondent 3:** I certainly have an issue with, I don't trust anything, research that's never going to be revealed . . . (FG3)

Many of the specialists suggested regular newsletters about Generation Scotland for those participating, both as good, ethical practice as well as a way of promoting trust and participation.

8.6.3 Governance, Regulation and Ownership

Although most participants talked about breaches of trust and the failure of processes and procedures to ensure confidentiality and prevent abuse, regulation and governance were also posited as solutions to issues of trust, fear and concern. All specialists felt that a clear set of rules, guidelines and protocols should be laid out and adhered to, offering stringent controls. There was a general view that governance of the database should be in the form of some kind of independent public body or trust. However, a variety of different oversight committees was suggested to ensure Generation Scotland is run satisfactorily. They included: a scientific review committee to decide what the data could be used for; a privacy/access committee to decide who should have access to the database (with rules for access made public on a Web site); various forms of ethical review committees; a review body, including members of the public. It was also argued that there needed to be a 'vetting and monitoring' of Generation Scotland that members of the public have access to. Whether this meant access to become part of that monitoring system or that the public could have access to their findings is unclear.

Many of the focus group respondents thought it important that the DNA database was 'publicly owned' (or controlled by public servants) or, at least, that there should be public or charitable representation and ethical oversight. Most felt Generation Scotland should be a public charity and that benefits should be community and publicly-based. For example, the Dementia Carers' group (FG10) emphasized 'control,' with the medical profession acting as 'gatekeepers.' They suggested that a 'trustee' representing the people who support Generation Scotland could control it, but not local councilors, politicians or pharmaceutical company personnel (those most distrusted it seems). Another group suggested that Generation Scotland could be an independent trust that 'owns' the database and licenses pharmaceutical companies to do work (FG3). In fact, several alternative solutions about who should control access were offered, including the Scottish Executive (government), the National Health Service or Universities.

Many of the participants turned to existing examples to draw parallels and identify appropriate models that might be adopted, such as those used by the Human Fertilisation and Embryology Authority (HFEA) and Scottish Blood Transfusion Service (SBTS). The Scottish Blood Transfusion Service, as an organisation, was viewed as trustworthy and one that Generation Scotland should emulate as a good ethical parallel—a proposal made by both specialists and publics' focus groups.

Despite varying ideas about who should be in control, the issue of control appeared vital in resolving ambivalence about access. Such sentiments were echoed in the following quotation from one specialist clinician involved in government:

> 'I would have said that GPs are most trusted by the public and it could well be this independent body would have to be made up of GPs who. . . . are trusted people by the public. We have to take into account that it would have to be an independent body, people who are not involved in this research so they don't see it as their livelihood being shall we say in jeopardy, or their research program. It's a very difficult one this and I think if politicians were involved in it they would not be trusted at all. If civil servants are involved they won't trust it at all. It's got to be people who they trust, who they feel there's no axe to grind and they're doing it for the good of the public, not for the good of their knighthoods, their money, everything else. It's a very difficult one this. And this is where I think these big data sets need to find some way forward . . . This has to be open, it mustn't be secret. The actual independent running of this should be open and actually open possibly to the public to attend. The public has to know that there is an independent body, made up of people they can trust that's open to the public and discusses what's going on.' (Clinician).

8.7   DISCUSSION AND CONCLUSION

This chapter has explored the way in which participants in a consultation process conducted at an early stage in the development of a genetic database for health research discussed the issues raised by such an endeavour. Notions of trust formed part of these discussions, both implicitly and explicitly. However, in line with previous research and current theorizing about trust, we should not be surprised that trust manifested in a differentiated way. Through discussion about issues such as participation in research, and access and control of data gathered and held, our findings suggest that mistrust and trust can sit quite comfortably alongside each other. Such specific subjects were embedded in wider matters about which participants also had opinions and experience. These latter issues related to 'a bigger picture,' so we saw, for example, fairly widespread support for the overall promise of science and the march of medical scientific progress. Moving one step further, we also found that aspects of Generation Scotland seemed to reinforce particular dimensions of trust, namely its national (i.e. Scottish) and therefore somewhat local nature.

Our findings also point to issues that challenge trust or shape mistrust, and again these can be understood to operate at different levels. On the one hand participants discussed the possibility, and even to some extent the inevitability, of 'big' breaches of trust, a stance borne of scepticism and culturally available experience (e.g., well-known cases of such breaches). On the other, these could be countered by examples of robust organizations and sound ethical practice (one example given was of the Scottish Blood Transfusion Service). This does indeed suggest that it is distant and abstract institutions that fail to engender trust. Other themes that suggest the cultural embeddedness of mistrust related to issues such as runaway science, being unable to control for 'rogues' or individual breaches and, as we have noted elsewhere (Haddow et al. 2007), concerns about access to information by commercial companies, for example insurance companies. There were some differences between participants here, with patient groups showing slightly more tolerance of pharmaceutical-company involvement in such research than others.

At the beginning of the chapter we raised questions about the so-called crisis of trust and the role of public consultation and engagement as an institutional response to such a perceived crisis. Our research reported here would suggest, as Wynne (2006) has noted, that the crisis of trust is somewhat of a myth. Certainly, mistrust does exist, but as noted above, it does so in the context of overall support for medical science and interestingly overall optimism about participating in the development of a genetic database that will only have long-term future benefits. Willingness to participate, then, seems to be occurring alongside specific concerns about control and access and a generalized scepticism and mistrust of large organizations, whether public or private. Participation can perhaps be conceptualized as both a token of trust (in this case in a local Scottish health-related genetic database) but also as token trust (because such participation does not seem to nullify concerns about potential breaches of trust).

Public consultation and engagement can, perhaps, go some way to resolving some of the dilemmas that this chapter has raised regarding trust and participation in genetic databases. So far, the research has helped identify key concerns about access and control that we have been able to feed back into the scientific and ethical management of Generation Scotland as well as to a wide audience, which may impact on policy. However, public consultation and engagement can raise yet more dilemmas for researchers such as ourselves. The process of engaging specialists and publics in research raises further issues of trust. Encouraging debate and reflection among participants in a consultation exercise, as we have done, for example, raises expectations about involvement and influence, and perhaps also means that trust has been placed in us to take issues forward and to feed issues back. There is still more to do, but we hope that, by exploring the nature of trust as expressed in the focus groups and interviews we conducted, we can contribute to the overall aim of Generation Scotland to create an ethically robust genetic database.

ACKNOWLEDGMENTS

We would like to thank all who gave up their time to participate in this study. We should also like to thank Ann Bruce, Claire Buré, Jane Ewins, Sarah Parry, Jennifer Speirs, and Eileen Mothersole for their help in setting up and conducting the focus groups and transcribing and analyzing the focus group tapes.

REFERENCES

Anderson, B. 1983. *Imagined Communities: Reflections on the Origin and Spread of Nationalism*. London: Verso.
Beck, U. 1997. *The Reinvention of Politics: Rethinking Modernity in the Global Social Order*. Cambridge: Cambridge Polity Press.
Brownlie, J., and A. Howson. 2005. 'Leaps of Faith' and MMR: An Empirical Study of Trust. *Sociology* 39 (2): 221–239.
Cunningham-Burley, S. 2006. Public Knowledge and Public Trust. *Community Genetics* 9 (3): 204–210.
Giddens, A. 1991. *Modernity and Self-Identity: Self and Society in the Late Modern Age*. Cambridge: Cambridge Polity Press.
Haddow, G., S. Cunningham-Burley, A. Bruce, and S. Parry. 2004. Generation Scotland Preliminary Consultation Exercise 2003–04: Public and Stakeholder Views from Focus Groups and Interviews 1–27). Edinburgh: ESRC INNOGEN Centre, the University of Edinburgh.
Haddow, G., G. Laurie, S. Cunningham-Burley, and K. Hunter. 2007. Tackling Community Concerns about Commercialization and Genetic Research: A Modest Interdisciplinary Proposal. *Social Science and Medicine* 64: 272–282.
House of Lords Select Committee on Science and Technology. *Science and Society, 3rd Report*. London HMSO 2000 [online]. Available from: <http://www.publications.parliament.uk/pa/ld199900/ldselect/ldsctech/38/3801.htm>
Irwin, A. 2006. The Politics of Talk: Coming to Terms with the New Scientific Governance. *Social Studies of Science* 36 (2): 299–320.
Jones, M., and B. Salter. 2003. The Governance of Human Genetics: Policy Discourse and Constructions of Public Trust. *New Genetics and Society* 22 (1): 21–41.
Kerr, A., S. Cunningham-Burley, and A. Amos. 1998. The New Genetics and Health: Mobilizing Lay Expertise. *Public Understanding of Science* 7 (1): 41–60.
Kerr, A., S. Cunningham-Burley, and R. Tutton. 2007. Shifting Subject Positions: Experts and Lay People in Public Dialogue. *Social Studies of Science* 37 (3): 385–411.
Khodyakov, D. 2007. Trust as a Process: A Three-Dimensional Approach. *Sociology* 41 (1): 115–132.
Lewis, D., and A. Weigert. 1985. Trust as a Social Reality. *Social Forces* 63 (4): 967–985.
Möllering, G. 2001. The Nature of Trust: From Georg Simmel to a Theory of Expectation, Interpretation and Suspension. *Sociology* 35 (2): 403–420.
Rose, H. 2001. *The Commodification of Bioinformation: The Icelandic Health Sector Database*. London: The Wellcome Trust.
Willis, R., and J. Wilsdon. 2004. *See Through Science*. Demos, London.

Wynne, B. 1996. May the Sheep Safely Graze? A Reflexive View of the Expert–Lay Divide, in *Risk, Environment and Modernity,* eds. S. Lash, B. Szerszynski, and B. Wynne (44–83). London: Sage.

Wynne, B. 2006. Public Engagement as a Means of Restoring Public Trust in Science—Hitting the Notes, but Missing the Music. *Community Genetics* 9: 211–220.

Box 1:

Focus Groups:

Cystic Fibrosis Patient Support Group FG1
Seniors' Group FG2
Cycling Club FG3
Breast Cancer Advocacy Group FG4
Rural Group FG5
Multiple Sclerosis Support Group FG6
Women's Hill Walking Club FG7
Sikh Women's Group FG8
Men's Choir FG9
Dementia Carer Support Group FG10

Specialists:

Bioethicist
Medical ethicist
Theologian
Public health professionals (3)
Clinical geneticist
Clinician/manager
Academic genetic scientists (2)
Industry scientist
Academic (genetics and insurance)
Information policy expert
Medical lawyers (2)
Lawyer
Patient data expert

---

9 The Elixir of Social Trust
Social Capital and Cultures of Challenge in Health Movements

Alex Law

9.1 INTRODUCTION

It is frequently claimed that enhanced well-being and health are among the most welcome side effects of social capital (Hawe and Shiel 2000). Over the past decade or so the concept of 'social capital' has become firmly established within Anglophone public health paradigms. Social capital is variously defined in terms of social norms, trust, reciprocity and interpersonal networks. For instance, Pierre Bourdieu defines social capital as 'the aggregate of the actual or potential resources which are linked to a durable network of more or less institutionalised relationships of mutual acquaintance or recognition' (2006, 110). Different thinkers emphasize various aspects of how the dimensions of social capital intersect to enable people to participate in and flourish through the collective structures of society (Portes 1998; Baron, et al. 2002). Without doubt the most influential theorist of social capital is the political scientist Robert D. Putnam (1993, 1995, 2000). His work is among the most cited in the English language social sciences and has been celebrated by both President Clinton in the United States and Prime Minister Tony Blair in the United Kingdom (Szreter 1999). Blair, for instance, eulogized Putnam's conception of social capital in his vision of the 'good community':

> 'As Robert Putnam argues . . . communities that are inter-connected are healthier communities. If we play football together, run parent-teacher associations together, sing in choirs or learn to paint together, we are less likely to want to cause harm to each other. Such inter-connected communities have lower crime, better education results, better care of the vulnerable.' (Blair 2002, 12–13).

As Putnam (2000) put it in his celebrated study *Bowling Alone*, a ten minute increase in commuting causes a 10 percent drop in community activity, whereas joining a club reduces by half the chances of dying next year. However, where supporting evidence for a positive relationship between social capital and improved health is weak, Putnam simply urges unquestioning support for the seductive message of social capital: 'Policy-makers should not have to wait for a couple of decades of detailed research before asking whether attentiveness to social capital might be worth their while' (2004, 15).

Though it may prove difficult to object to such wholesome images of neighbourly trust, participation and public virtue in public health studies, social capital tends to be undertheorized and Putnam's psychological, economistic and communitarian premises accepted uncritically (Navarro 2002; Fine 2001). Despite its routine usage and positive associations, social capital remains a profoundly contested term.

In the light of Putnam's unrivalled influence over the wide circulation of social capital as a health discourse, this chapter aims to critically examine his conception of the role of trust within the social capital paradigm. In the process, criticisms of Putnam's assumptions about the relationship between social trust and health are advanced, not least because the positive association with health attributed to social capital is *not* uniformly supported by other research findings (Lynch, et al. 2000; Lynch, et al. 2001; Chavez, Kemp and Harris 2004). Putnam's notion of social trust is further contested in this chapter through consideration of the role played by social movements, specifically ones concerned with health issues. Drawing from a case study of a local grassroots campaign against cellular phone towers (or masts as they are known in the U.K.) I show how the idea of 'cultures of challenge' in health movements disputes Putnam's notion of social trust as essentially consensual and prepolitical. Although this case study did not begin with an explicit focus on questions of trust and mistrust, they soon emerged as crucial variables. Stakeholders were highly conscious of being seen as 'trustworthy' even while they played a tactical game to outmanoeuvre their opponents. This reflects the shifting scales of trust characteristic of modernity: from those inscribed in face-to-face community relationships to abstract and unseen sociotechnical systems, populated by anonymous experts.

Given the paradoxical role that 'trust' played in this public health campaign, my main focus in this chapter is to explicate the varying role played by (dis)trust in social capital and (inter)personal flourishing. Health inequalities cannot be detached from the wider patterning of social relations (Kawachi and Kennedy 1997). Such inequalities not only condition positive feelings of autonomy, connectedness and agency, they also socially shape relative degrees of mistrust, atomisation and suspicion. Trust, therefore, may prove a more ambivalent feature of interpersonal flourishing than is generally assumed in communitarian models of social capital.

9.2   BOWLED OVER: PUTNAM AND SOCIAL TRUST

In his best-selling book *Bowling Alone: The Collapse and Revival of American Community*, Putnam (2000) diagnoses the national and personal malaise of American society in terms of the steady disintegration of social capital.

This has been accompanied by long-term trends in worsening indices of mental illness, depression and suicide, which Putnam correlates to falling levels of civic engagement. Suicide rates are not borne uniformly across U.S. society but have a generational dimension; suicide is less common among older cohorts and more prevalent among younger ones. Older people born in the 1920s and 1930s form what Putnam (2000, 262) calls the 'well-integrated long civic generation' who are active in more organizations than younger people born in the 1970s and 1980s, the so-called 'X Generation.' The symptoms of personal malaise—headaches, indigestion and sleeplessness—has increased sharply for the under-thirties cohort, but they have declined for the over-sixties 'civic generation.' As the older civic generation with a high-trust quotient declines as a percentage of the population, they are replaced by a younger generation that exhibits much lower levels of trust, leading to a decline in civility and civic activism and a rise in sociopathic conduct, such as 'road rage' and general noncooperation with civic duties, such as refusing to return census forms. This leads Putnam to conflate causal relations of social processes for statistical correlations of demographic change: '*Though all the evidence is not in,* it is hard to believe that the generational decline in social connectedness and the concomitant generational increase in suicide, depression and malaise are unrelated' (Putnam 2000, 265, emphasis added). In the absence of supporting data, he posits an unambiguous association between civic engagement and personal well-being, '*whether or not* generational differences in social capital fully account for age-related differences in suicide rates' (2000, 262, emphasis added). Putnam firmly accents voluntary participation and interpersonal association as a vehicle for certain kinds of improved health outcomes, but less polarized health outcomes in society depend, at least in part, on a more egalitarian redistribution of material resources (Das 2006; Kawachi and Kennedy 1997).

Social capital advocates such as Putnam claim that the concept can be made to explain, measure and remedy almost anything, in any realm or context, from twelfth century Europe to twenty-first century Africa. For instance, in his foreword to the World Bank's study of social capital, Putnam, outlines the concept in unbridled Promethean terms:

> 'While early work had focused primarily on governance, macroeconomic rates of growth, and (in closely related) work school performance and job placement, we now are beginning to see how *social capital can influence everything* from infant mortality rates to solid waste management to communal violence.' (2000, xxii, emphasis added).

Social capital functions as a conceptual *deus ex machina*. It can be made to explain any 'thing' that appears to be broken down and needs to be fixed back in place, ranging from the sick, the poor, the criminal, the corrupt, the (dys)functional family, schooling, community life, work and organisation, democracy and governance, collective action, transitional societies, economies, and institutions (Fine 2001, 190). Moreover, social capital depends on an orthodox notion of 'capital,' deepening the colonization of the social sciences by economistic discourses (Fine 2001; Law and Mooney, 2006). For instance, Putnam sympathetically quotes Nobel-prize economist Kenneth Arrow on the economics of trust: 'It can be plausibly argued that much of the economic backwardness in the world can be explained by the lack of mutual confidence' (1993, 170). Specifically, social phenomena like interpersonal relations of trust are thereby reduced to mathematical formulae. Too often the assumed relationship between trust, networks, reciprocity and health in survey data mistakes a statistical correspondence of inessential correlation for prior processes of social causation (Foley and Edwards 1998).

Echoing an older theme from the functionalist sociology of Emile Durkheim, social atomization and 'rampant individualism' are held by Putnam to simultaneously account for low trust, weak civic engagement and the malaise afflicting younger Americans. Conversely, social capital possesses 'remarkable health benefits': 'The more integrated we are with our community, the less likely we are to experience colds, heart attacks, strokes, cancer, depression, and premature death of all sorts' (Putnam 2000, 326). Putnam advances a number of hypotheses to explain the positive role played by social cohesion in health outcomes. First, dense social networks reduce unnecessary stress and suffering through the practical support they provide for all manner of social need, from relatively minor, day-to-day requirements such as borrowing sugar from neighbours to helping individuals to cope with personal loss. Second, socially cohesive communities can reinforce healthy norms and hazard-reducing conduct, whereas social isolation tends to encourage health-damaging behaviour like alcoholism. Third, well-organized communities are also more able to effectively organise and articulate political demands to defend or improve local health services. Finally, social capital may have positive biochemical effects, enhancing bodily resistance to disease and illness, whereas social isolation may precipitate ill-health.

By enhancing trustful social relations, social capital is therefore deemed an independent variable affecting the *quantity* of life, how long we live, as well as the *quality* of life, profoundly shaping the character of social interaction. Civic activism is not only good for the soul and conscience of volunteers, for Putnam it is literally a life saver:

'If you belong to no groups but decide to join one, you cut your risk of dying over the next year in half. If you smoke and belong to no groups it's a toss-up statistically whether you should stop smoking or start joining. These findings are in some ways heartening: it's easier to join a group than to lose weight, exercise regularly, or quit smoking.' (2000, 331).

The erosion of social capital has equally detrimental effects. Geographical distance, even when mediated by communication technologies, cannot reproduce the therapeutic qualities of face-to-face social interaction. Along with income and marriage, Putnam claims that face-to-face civic engagement raises the 'happiness quotient,' the feeling of well-being and contentment, whereas poverty, solitariness, and civic disengagement reinforce misanthropy, nihilism and anomie. Heightened financial insecurity, even among more affluent groups, overlaps with social disconnectedness to produce a loss of trust, autonomy, control and belonging. As the lubricant of trust evaporates, social conduct becomes increasingly codified and formalized in contracts, litigation, audit and reporting cultures, and increased state regulation (Putnam 2000, 145).

9.2.1   Trustworthiness and Social Capital

At the core of Putnam's conception of social capital is trust or, rather, 'trustworthiness.' For Putnam, this refers to the general state of 'social trust' enjoyed by a community. Social trust is founded on two basic premises—norms of reciprocity and civic networks (Putnam 1993, 171). First, norms ease social intercourse and cooperation through either immediate, tangible exchanges or the 'generalized reciprocity' of deferred exchanges that promise to be repaid, if at all, at some future point. It is the latter, 'generalized' form of reciprocity that is crucial for Putnam as it prevents narrow self-interest from eroding the bases of social exchange. Individuals flourish in conditions of social trust due to what might be called their 'altruistic self-interest' in generalized relations of reciprocity. Trustworthiness leads to altruistic conduct such as good neighbourliness and honesty, which, in the long run, helps to establish mutual honesty and moral security as a generalized condition that benefits each and all. As the popular maxim puts it, 'one good turn deserves another.' 'Good turns' become mutually reinforcing until they cannot be separated from everyday activism and trustful expectations: 'The causal arrows among civic involvement, reciprocity, honesty and social trust are as tangled as well-tossed spaghetti' (Putnam, 2000, 137).

'Generalized reciprocity' represents the fundamental principle of social capital. Such a principle is only present when social trust is sufficiently widespread or 'generalized' that it determines the social atmosphere within which everyday exchanges occur. Not only is social trust a public good in its own right, it is also socially and economically efficient because the 'moral community' that it depends upon lowers what economists call 'transaction costs' (Fukyama 1995). These extra costs are incurred when social (and economic) exchanges need to be formalized or mediated by a third party due to the low levels of trust in the relationship. Hence social trust becomes a valued 'community asset,' not an attribute of individuals:

> 'A society that relies on generalized reciprocity is more efficient than a distrustful society, for the same reason that money is more efficient than barter. Honesty and trust lubricate the inevitable frictions of life.' (Putnam 2000, 135).

If Putnam identifies social capital as having health-enhancing properties then, inversely, the 'artificial trust' represented by formal instruments of social regulation such as contractual arrangements are assumed to possess debilitating effects for health as well as economic efficiency. However, as Putnam further argues, should individuals engage in unconditional trust in a generally untrustworthy social setting such as a discriminatory workplace or a corrupt boardroom then they are merely acting as gullible dupes.

Second, trustworthiness is a condition of social networks—not a property of individual psychology. Involved here are different intensities of trust ranging from what Putnam calls 'thin trust' in the relations of mutuality between 'generalized others' of casual acquaintance to the 'thick trust' embedded in dense social networks, where interaction is routine and frequent enough to ensure that trustworthiness is a positively assumed social norm. 'Thick trust' broadly corresponds to 'bonding' forms of exclusive social capital found in dense networks such as ethnically homogenous enclaves. 'Thin trust' is closer to 'bridging' forms of inclusive social capital that link heterogeneous groups through what Mark Granovetter (1973) called 'the strength of weak ties.' These different intensities of social trust may have direct consequences for community activism and health. 'Bonding' through the 'strong ties' of dense social networks can exclude outsiders; make excessive claims on group members; enforce conformity; and its norms can impose lower aspirations. Health may in fact suffer under restrictive community norms, as in postwar affluent suburban communities where women's possibilities for autonomy suffered under received patriarchal norms. In any case, the relationship is far from uni-causal and their effects multifarious:

> 'In one context, strong friendship networks of peers can increase the risk of smoking, drinking or use of illicit drugs, while in a different situation these same sort of links may decrease the risk of suicide. Tight networks among the members of anti-immigrant, racist or plutocratic political parties, semi-clandestine business organizations such as the Trilateral Commission or the World Trade Organization, or nonelected, unaccountable international financial institutions like the World Bank may in fact increase health risks for other members of the population.' (Muntaner, Lynch et al. 2001, 219).

Others extol the efficacy of slack, informal social coalitions and return to Granovetter's (1973) emphasis on 'loose ties.' In conditions of 'thin trust' between generalized others the assumption of reciprocity holds until it is broken through distrust experienced in the casual associations of social milieu. Some groups offer their thin trust more unconditionally than others. Hence, the poor and the oppressed, who in the past have been on the receiving end of bad faith, humiliation and discrimination, according to Putnam, tend to be more distrustful of the 'generalized other' and seek solace in defensive communitarian forms of bonded social capital as described above. This dense form of social capital appears to have fewer health benefits for neighbourhoods than the loose ties of bridging social capital (Cattell 2001). Putnam also views small towns as more trusting than large cities, even though large cities may be places of greater freedom and liberty. However, others dispute the evidential basis of a direct correspondence between associational density and trust (see Milner 2002).

9.3 TRUST AND POLITICAL CULTURE

In a further echo of functionalist sociology, trust and contentment appear to be more thoroughly valued by Putnam than competing virtues like freedom and dissent. Social capital enjoyed in civic association becomes a way to evade difficult, oppositional and antagonistic political activism. Putnam discusses trust in the communitarian form of civic engagement, but others stress the prior political, institutional and legal framework of civic activism (Milner 2002). Indeed social trust as a measure of collective sensibility is profoundly shaped by national cultures. For example, interpersonal trust may be more important for collective activity in highly individualized cultures like that of the United States than in more collective cultures such as those of Canada and Scandinavia, where group rights and an enlarged role for the state prevails, perhaps diminishing the need for explicit norms to regulate interpersonal conduct.

National systems of authority help determine the quality as well as the extent of social trust. As Putnam (2000, 136) notes, only a saint or a fool can possibly flourish through trustful conduct where conditions of generalised mendacity have established social mistrust as the governing norm. Such 'chronic mendacity' is precisely what some see as accurately describing the contemporary public relations cynicism of government and corporate interests that lies behind market-driven, neoliberal policy regimes such as that of the United Kingdom (Leys 2000; Marquand 2004). It is claimed that the public interest in trust-based communication systems and public services in the United Kingdom has been seriously eroded by elite deceit, 'spin' and the (mis)management of the public agenda through the mobilisation of duplicitous language around warfare, corporate interests and political debate (Fairclough 2000; Miller and Dinan 2007). Repeated episodes of communicative cynicism in the United Kingdom, from the BSE crisis to the 'sexed-up' intelligence dossier that helped launch the Iraq war, it is argued, erodes public trust in traditional authority. Furthermore, what Richard Sennett calls 'the culture of the new capitalism' (2006, 68) of abrupt changes in institutional personnel and organizational structures imposed from above and from outside, undermines the extended time frames and network stability needed to generate and reproduce tacit reciprocity and mutuality.

Indeed, in the United Kingdom since the 1980s there has been a marked decline in political trust in politicians, political parties and governmental institutions (The Power Inquiry 2006). Such trends are especially evident in younger cohorts. However, associational membership and civic engagement remain vibrant in the United Kingdom, and within this wide base of voluntary activity, grassroots activists appear to enjoy higher morale, self-confidence and commitment. Low levels of political trust in formal institutions are not only a result of more cynical public-relations politics but seem also to be part of a wider alienation arising from the hollowing out of state authority behind market-driven imperatives (Leys 2000). Such shifts have produced less deferential observance of hierarchically organized social and political power and are consistent with 'do-it-yourself' lifestyle values of self-esteem and self-actualization (The Power Inquiry 2006, 64).

In Scotland, people still tend to exhibit relatively high levels of trust in their immediate neighbours and show a general social trust in complete strangers (Paterson 2002, 9). These levels of trust are linked to a higher propensity to get involved in associations of various kinds. Unlike Putnam's analysis of the 'civic generation' in the United States, in Scotland no discernible demographic trend is apparent. As Paterson concludes: 'it is clear that in Scotland, networks are associated with norms and trust. It does seem useful and not too simplifying to refer to the whole nexus of trust, norms and networks by the singular term social capital' (2002, 19). From Paterson's analysis of social attitude survey data, social trust was further related to low levels of cynicism, something that perhaps ought to hold true by definition. However, high levels of trust, strong norms and dense networks are strongly related to affluent groups in Scotland who subscribe to a more authoritarian ideology. On the other hand, weak social trust in Scotland is associated with dissatisfaction with the U.K. state and translates into support to decentralise power away from the London Parliament to the devolved Scottish Parliament.

9.3.1   Trust and Community

Paterson's analysis of social attitudes in Scotland seems to lend support to claims made by Putnam on behalf of a strong relationship between social capital, trust and politics. Where institutional social capital and national political cultures tend towards corrupt, unresponsive, remote or draconian forms of government the public health of the community suffers accordingly as the 'bridge' to effective political activism through participation, public voice and autonomy is withdrawn. Mistrust of community leaders, private corporations and government becomes more widespread due to a lack of accountability and effective political dialogue. For example, this was found to be the case in the urban redevelopment of East Baltimore, one of the least healthy communities in the United States, where political disenfranchisement from the redevelopment process and physical displacement only exacerbated mental disorder, chronic illness and premature death in the community (Gomez and Muntaner 2005).

Other studies have shown a relationship between (mis)trust and neighbourhood mortality rates (Lochner et al. 2003). A study of two disadvantaged communities in Sydney, Australia, found that of the various components of social capital—neighbourhood attachment, sense of personal safety, feelings of trust and reciprocity, support networks, local engagement, and personal attachment to the locality—only 'trust' was positively associated with self-reported health and that 'no other components of social capital were significant in explaining health variances in these disadvantaged neighbourhoods' (Chavez et al. 2004, S2, 33). More important for explaining health variances in this study were well-known structural characteristics of class, age, gender and housing type.

In his earlier study of the logic of democratic activism in Italy, Putnam (1993, 167) argued that regions which embed 'civic virtue' in high 'stocks' of social capital—that is, dense networks of reciprocal social relations, norms and trust—more efficiently facilitate mutual cooperation for the greater good. The good community causes the successful economy and the powerful state rather than vice versa: 'Social capital, as embodied in horizontal networks of civic engagement, bolsters the performance of the polity and the economy, rather than the reverse: strong society, strong economy; strong society, strong state' (Putnam 1993, 176). Though abundant in northern Italy, Putnam found social capital lacking in the south. Instead southern Italy was marked by traditions of parochialism, distrust and disengagement. Thus entire regions become prisoners of a culture of distrust, with negative implications for health outcomes.

The idea that national and regional cultures of (dis)trust determine the voluntary activism of members of a community rests, however, on a tautology. It conflates culture, social process, social agency and social outcomes in a whirlpool of conceptual confusion. It fails to show that the possession of social capital—trust (culture) and civic engagement (agency)—is in some sense logically prior to the benign outcomes it bestows on group members. Indeed, Putnam seems uncertain about the direction of the relationship, at times extolling voluntary activity as prior to social trust but elsewhere claiming an antecedent role for social trust, which is already made available as a property of deeply embedded local customs. In any case, social trust has *not* been found to be the primary determinant of civic engagement and cooperation, leading some critics to argue that 'use of generalized social trust as the focus of attention in political scientists' work is a dead end' (Foley and Edwards cited in Milner 2002, 21).

Social trust thus becomes both the circular cause and effect of healthy civic communities: Social capital is present wherever civic engagement can be observed and vice versa. Indeed, Putnam's strong identification of social capital with social trust insufficiently delineates other forms of trust outside communitarian notions. Communitarian 'thick trust' and civic 'thin trust' refer to interpersonal or 'horizontal trust,' which may directly contradict 'vertical trust,' understood as trust in hierarchies, political leaders and institutions. Putnam assumes an inverse relationship between vertical and horizontal trust and denies that a vertical network can ever sustain social trust and cooperation (1993, 174). As such Putnam opens up an ideological line of attack on 'vertical institutions' like the welfare state. For instance, he ignores the political and social history of the National Health Service (NHS) in the United Kingdom, which was created as a vertical institution precisely to redress the *failure* of civic, horizontal relations of mutuality and voluntarism to sustain an adequate provision of health and social care. He also neglects the widespread sense of vertical trust in the NHS shown by the U.K. electorate in numerous Social Attitudes Surveys, an attachment that deepened when the NHS appeared to be threatened by various U.K. governments during the 1980s and 1990s. Rather than blind trust, this can be put down to what Milner (2002) calls the high levels of 'civic literacy'—the knowledge and capacity of the populace to make sense of their political world. Political or civic literacy expressed in the United Kingdom as a popular commitment to relatively egalitarian outcomes in the distribution of health-sustaining resources provides a more solid foundation to understanding the relationship between the culture of social trust and the agency of civic engagement.

9.4   THE CHALLENGE OF SOCIAL MOVEMENTS

Particularly important to the civic and physical health of any society is the role played by various kinds of politically literate social movements. Social movements create social capital by producing new conditions for mutual reciprocity through extending the reach of existing social networks and fostering new senses of group identity and belonging. Only movements rooted locally in direct face-to-face accountability, rather than national, large-scale bureaucratic movements, represent the kinds of interpersonal solidarity and intense civic commitment that Putnam calls social capital. National organizations, such as the British Labour Party, that rely on a passive membership and a centralized full-time staff, cannot in any meaningful sense be said to be building the health-enhancing social capital advocated by Putnam. As he pithily put it: 'Citizenship by proxy is an oxymoron' (2000, 160). Yet Putnam is curiously negligent about the actual ideological content of social movements. He views them as an unalloyed public good just so long as they invigorate civic engagement:

> 'Whether among gays marching in San Francisco or evangelicals praying together on the Mall or, in an earlier era, autoworkers downing tools in Flint, the act of collective protest itself creates enduring bonds of solidarity . . . In short, social movements with grassroots involvement both embody and produce social capital.' (Putnam 2000, 153).

In the United States, Putnam claims, it is much easier for evangelical right-wing movements to mobilize grassroots activity in ways in which 'progressive' social movements like the national environmental organizations such as Greenpeace do not and perhaps cannot. Campaigns such as the latter rely on the media-led, symbolic capital of global political objectives rather than the local activity and mobilisation of high social capital, typically undertaken by older protesters. On the other hand, we have also seen the resurgence of youthful 'progressive' activism across the United States and Europe, in the antiglobalisation protests in Seattle in 1999, the opposition to the Iraq war, and the struggles of working-class Hispanic-Americans over low pay and immigration rights. Here the problem is Putnam's nostalgia for 'mainstream' activism. Now that the social eruptions of the 1960s have dissipated or been assimilated, as he put it, 'The tensile strength of the newer organizations is much weaker' (Putnam 2000, 158). The rise and decline of rank and file, radical grassroots movements of the 1960s and 1970s seems like a minor interlude between longer phases of the dominance of conservative social capital (Law and Mooney 2006). Putnam rather arbitrarily focuses on what might be termed high trust 'cultures of conformism' but neglects or dismisses other forms of activism in the 'cultures of challenge' (Scrambler and Kelleher 2006), as evident in campaigns to defend services, jobs and amenities and environmental and anticapitalist protest against systemic inequalities. Cultures of conformism attend to the apparently innocuous activities that pose little threat to powerful interests. This can include providing charitable services to the disadvantaged as much as participating in sports clubs. Because no challenge to structural interests is involved, it evinces no direct political implications.

9.4.1 Health Movements

One way that a vigorous civic culture remains viable is in the emergence of social movements around health issues, in defence of welfare services as well as wider environmental and political matters. Health has become a primary detonator of grassroots movements. The scope of health movements, however, needs to include not only those directly concerned with medical knowledge and practice but also movements that challenge medical, technological and scientific authority indirectly. These take in campaigns around perceived public health hazards where the focus might include private corporations, planners, politicians and scientific experts. Participation in oppositional health campaigns can become empowering in ways that social capitalists like Putnam fail to anticipate:

> '[Campaign movements] have emerged as part of a *culture of challenge* in which people are increasingly able and prepared to contest expert systems. Through the confidence they gain as movement participants, whether they attend local groups or simply see themselves, via media debates, as part of an 'imagined' one, they feel they acquire

the confidence to interrogate doctors and treatment options.' (Scrambler and Kelleher 2006, 229).

While the environmental justice movement has played a significant part in the raising of health consciousness, perhaps the key exemplar of this shift has been the Women's Health Movement in the United States (Morgen 2002), which has helped democratize health issues and challenge medico-centrism. Health social movements, like the Women's Health Movement, are concerned with 'collective challenges to medical policy and politics, belief systems, research and practice that include an array of formal and informal organisations, supporters, networks of co-operation, and media' (Brown et al. 2004, 52).

Health-related movements have been classified into three basic ideal types (Brown et al. 2004). First, 'health access movements' mobilize around improving the access to, and provision of, services. Second, 'constituency-based movements' mobilize specific social strata in definite localities to redress health inequalities arising from class, gender, ethnicity or sexuality. Third, 'embodied health movements' mobilize around disability and illness and contest the biomedical model of health conceived as a positive science. In the case of our study of the local anti-phone mast movement it is both a constituency-based health movement—it contests the siting of health hazards in a particular community on the basis of social milieu and gender—and it is also an embodied movement—concerned with the potential negative health effects on the biological bodies of local adults and children.

Health-related movements are further differentiated by the methods and goals they pursue. On the one hand, advocacy-based movements exhibit high levels of trust in rational dialogue and work within the dominant medical paradigm in order to have lay concerns accepted within expert knowledge systems (Barnes, Newman and Sullivan 2007). On the other hand, activist-based movements have lower levels of trust in the rationality and responsiveness of expert knowledge systems, employ direct action to challenge dominant scientific and medical paradigms and cultivate wider democratic participation in decision making. In both forms of advocacy and activism, health movements perform as 'boundary movements' that 'blur the edges' between experts and lay people (Brown et al. 2004). Scrambler and Kelleher (2006) build a more precise typology of the 'mobilizing potentials' of health-related movements ranging from: 'rights' as demanded by disability activists; 'users' such as mental health users; 'campaigns' based on a single issue such as local pollution; 'identity' politics like third wave feminism; to 'politics' based on national organisations like Greenpeace. Such movements undertake such 'boundary work' to redetermine the authoritative character of expert knowledge systems, with the aim of exposing the internal validation processes of positive science to lay challenge and debate (Gieryn 1983).

9.5 NO2TETRA AS A HEALTH MOVEMENT

A local campaign, NO2TETRA, was initiated in 2003 in the towns and villages of northeast Fife, Scotland, to oppose perceived health risks from the siting of mast antennae and ancillary equipment for a national police radio system, Terrestrial Trunked Radio (TETRA). Research was carried out into the development of the campaign by attending public meetings, collecting campaign and promotional literature, analysing press cuttings and conducting semistructured interviews with campaigners, the company PR spokesperson, the chairperson of the local authority planning committee and the local journalist covering the story (see Law and McNeish 2007).

Planning conflicts emerged over potential health risks, such as cancers, headaches, skin disorders and sleep deprivation, derived from mast emissions of microwave radiation, even though the scientific evidence suggests that radiation from masts could be considerably lower than emissions from mobile handsets (Stewart 2000). Attempts to assuage the health concerns of local people by the telecommunications industry failed, and planners confronted a lack of community trust. Moreover, mistrust of experts was prevalent from the perspective of a fairly affluent, semirural community, with high levels of loose bridging ties combined with localised bonds. For some commentators, 'health-obsessed' activists merely act as 'risk entrepreneurs,' disseminating irrational fears through undermining the credibility of scientific authority as tainted by corporate and political interests. As Burgess (2004, 121–122) put it in his study of public fears of cellular phones: 'With a heightened sense of the importance of health, we are liable at least to consider any claim that harm may be posed, from even the most apparently innocuous source.'

Our case study shows how 'campaigning' developed mobilizing potential (Scrambler and Kelleher 2006) as a local protest against experts operating in line with the economic and political imperatives of corporate rationality (Law and McNeish 2007). Not only do medical professionals face a 'culture of challenge': in our research, scientific, political, and media experts were challenged by the mobilising potential of local women in particular. These women emerged as knowledgeable social actors able to shift between different fields of activity from holding public meetings, writing press releases, phoning round key actors, studying and retranslating expert literature into lay discourses, organising protests and dealing with the authorities (c.f. Barnes et al. 2007). They gained in confidence as the campaign spread into the public sphere of media comment and political discourse in the Scottish Parliament.

Activists, moved to initiate something, organized public meetings with scientific experts, corporate spokespeople and politicians, placed stories in the local and national press, organised demonstrations, and successfully placed a petition before the Scottish Parliament. In so doing, their perceived threat of phone mast hazard became a contentious public issue. In the process, the practical activity of activists represented a breach in the routines of everyday life, even where it was locally based and planted firmly in the soil of bonded relations of community. An important finding was that the campaign, like many others, appeared to have all the hallmarks of high social capital insofar as it was based on trustful horizontal relations generated across social networks of local acquaintances. Yet, though local campaigners maintained strong trusting relations among themselves, they simultaneously deeply distrusted the authority and motives of scientific experts, officials and politicians.

9.5.1   Selfhood and Trust

From the first public meeting that they organized in a Fife market town in April 2003, activists' own sense of selfhood was altered. By their public act of opposition they became different kinds of neighbours, friends, acquaintances, colleagues—ones who now needed to advance reasoned justifications for activism, formulated in such ways that were persuasive at least to their immediate social milieu. The shift into public forms of activism has an effect on implicit cultures of social trust and interpersonal well-being. This crossing of the line into activism, under the impact of a collective shock, Barker (1999, 23), is akin to Durkheim's notion of 'collective effervescence' and the role it plays in opening up overt forms of conflict and protest:

> 'Collective action has an element of disturbance of ritual, the dishonouring of power and challenging of existing structure. A decision for collective action sets going a chain of incidents, decisions, counter-responses ad mobilisations which together provide the inner temporal narrative of an 'event' as it moves from 'breach' to 'crisis' to eventual outcome.'

By sharpening the cleavage between communities and experts and by extending the public sphere away from corporate domination, an effective 'culture of challenge' helped NO2TETRA to generalize and reorder relations of trustworthiness around health-related issues in ways that communitarian models of social capital seek to avoid. The opening up of such an oppositional frame lessened the risk of activists being coopted by planners as can happen in organised policy forums (Barnes et al. 2007), though some group members were frustrated by the overwhelming focus of the campaign on media coverage and constitutional processes rather than on direct action tactics (Law and McNeish 2007). Such 'cultures of challenge' based on high levels of intracommunity trust and low levels of trust in experts counters Giddens' (1990) claim that modernity progressively supplants local, interpersonal relations of social trust with unconditional trust in abstract expert systems transcending time and space. Yet this needs to be qualified, as alternative sources of expertise are often called upon in 'cultures of challenge.' As MacKenzie put it, 'Disbelief in one set of experts' knowledge claims is often belief in those of others, in those of environmental groups such as Greenpeace, for example, rather than in those of biotechnology companies such as Monsanto' (2001, 9).

Yet this sweeping analysis neglects the specific, shifting balance between the bonds of strong ties and the bridging between weak ones involved in any social movement. Social movements and social trust are mutually reinforcing in dynamic ways (Diani and McAdam 2003). A health movement rooted in preexisting strong ties based on preformed mutuality and trust needs to extend its reach to mobilize wider constituencies in order to enhance its political effectiveness. Indeed, a movement based solely on contingent and diverse networks may lack the tensile strength that trust relations provided for NO2TETRA. Where trust is weak or lacking, fissures in the movement open up. Mistrust in small campaign groups inhibit further mobilization. In order to avoid potential fault lines, NO2TETRA combined strong and weak ties, mediated by what Olemacher (1996) calls 'social relays' between the homogeneity and heterogeneity of overlapping networks. As Edwards and McCarthy (2004, 627) put it: 'To be effective in mobilization, social relays must strike a balance between a broad base of weak ties that tap into the heterogeneity of society and a "critical mass" of relatively homogenous subnetworks among activists and leaders, especially at the outset of mobilization.' (2004, 627).

Strong social ties in a community-based health campaign will attempt to extend beyond immediate circles of activists whose trust and reliability is already established. Not only trusted 'friends' need to be recruited but also wider constituencies of 'strangers' (Jasper and Poulsen 1995). 'Moral shocks' experienced within a community affected by a decision taken externally help to diffuse feelings of both 'inner trust' locally and 'outer mistrust' of experts and their institutional bases. Moral shocks are taken up interpersonally and made sense of as a unified grievance. As Jasper (1997, 107) put it:

> 'Positive feelings toward one's home and surroundings, coupled with strong negative affect toward a proposal that seems to threaten these, are common raw materials for a protest. Activists must weave together a moral, cognitive and emotional package of attitudes. By framing the problem as, say, "big business" or "instrumentalism" they suggest a moral judgement: disregard or abuse of humans by bureaucracy.' (1997, 107).

NO2TETRA campaigners strongly felt that the siting of phone masts in their vicinity, accompanied by the loss of protective shelter in homes and public buildings such as hospitals and schools, was invasive. Unconditional trust in the verifiable safety of the technology was withheld by the campaigners, which led directly to a lack of trust in the company, the local authorities and the scientists who demanded that their reassurances be taken in good faith. Feelings of vertical distrust propelled the campaign outwards, bridging towards 'strangers' in a new configuration of social trust.

9.6   SOCIAL TRUST, SOCIAL CAPITAL
AND HEALTH INEQUALITIES

This analysis of NO2TETRA reveals something of the 'thickness' of trust, networks and reciprocity within a health movement and avoids the risk of reifying trust as a universal property outside of the study of particular milieu. In particular, the study teases out some deficits in Putnam's account of the relation between social capital and trust.

Putnam tends to make conservative assumptions about a world that has been lost, where more recent changes in family formation—especially increasing family diversity, increasing lone parent families, absent fathers—have contributed to a deficit in social capital (Edwards 2004). But in the NO2TETRA movement, women from a range of family structures were able to lead and build oppositional activism campaign that depended on horizontal forms of trust at a community level and vertical forms of distrust at government and corporate level. Moreover, this health movement developed from a community not particularly noted for its activism or oppositional politics, though a clear sense of 'community' was conveyed throughout our observations and interviews. There was no need, in other words, for activism to overcome what Putnam views as community decline and growing individualism, where social trust needs to be restored through civic engagement.

Further, Putnam makes little of how social trust and civic engagement might reverse the vicious cycle of poverty, deprivation and illness. Indeed, although the accent on reciprocity and networks may be useful for understanding interpersonal relations in more or less stable, bounded communities, there is little discussion in the social capital literature of how socioeconomic inequalities and gendered networks shape health outcomes (Molyneux 2002). Yet, more than trust is needed before health, or any other social good, is made dependent on social capital. In certain situations it may be entirely understandable, for instance, if individuals and communities withdraw their trust from certain kinds of authorized experts, as the NO2TETRA case shows. It is not obviously the case that even high levels of social capital will generate trust in expert knowledge of health hazards. And in terms of causation it is tautological to claim that social capital enables certain successful groups to 'succeed' while the absence of such resources accounts for the 'failure' of groups whose health is failed by an iniquitous social structure (Muntaner et al. 2001).

9.7   CONCLUSION: THE POLITICS OF
SOCIAL CAPITAL AND TRUST

An attraction of social capital is that it provides a rationale for reducing the scope of the welfare state despite the persistence of market failure.

Politics and economics are reduced to sociocultural networks of association, which, in turn, are reduced to an idealist social psychology. As Muntaner et al. argued about the impact of Third Way social capital for understanding public health:

> 'Social capital presents itself as an alternative to materialist structural inequalities (class, gender and race) by bringing to the forefront of social epidemiology an appealing common sense idealist social psychology to which everyone can relate (e.g., good relations with your community are good for your health). The use of social capital invokes a romanticised view of communities without social conflict (e.g., neo-Tocquevillian nineteenth century associationalism) and favours an idealist psychology over a psychology connected to both material resources and social structure.' (2001, 107).

By advancing an idealist social psychology, the idea of social capital helps the weak and the vulnerable to help themselves, just as Baron von Munchhausen dragged himself and his horse out of the mire by his own hair. Health movements like NO2TETRA illustrate some of the limits to social capital and suggest a need for a more refined approach to the relationship between social structure, activism, health and social trust.

REFERENCES

Barker, C. 1999. Empowerment and resistance: "Collective effervescence" and other accounts. In *Transforming Poltics: Power and Resistance*, eds. P. Bagguley and J. Hern. Basingstoke: Macmillan Press.

Barnes, M., J. Newman, and H. Sullivan. 2007. *Power, Participation and Political Renewal: Case Studies in Public Participation*. Bristol: Policy Press.

Baron, S., J. Field, and T. Schuller, eds. 2002. *Social Capital: Critical Perspectives*. Oxford: Oxford University Press.

Blair, T. 2002. New Labour and community. *Renewal*, 10 (2): 9–14.

Bourdieu, P. 2006. The forms of capital. In *Education, Globalization & Social Change*, eds. H. Lauder, P. Brown, J. Dillaborough, and A. H. Halsey. Oxford: Oxford University Press.

Brown, P., S. Zavestoski, S. McCormick, B. Mayer, R. Morello-Frosch, and R. G. Altman. 2004. Embodied health movements: New approaches to social movements in health. *Sociology of Health & Illness* 26 (1): 50–80.

Burgess, A. 2004. *Cellular Phones, Public Fears, and a Culture of Precaution*. Cambridge: Cambridge University Press.

Cattell, V. 2001. Poor people, poor places, and poor health: The mediating role of social networks and social capital. *Social Science and Medicine* 52 (10): 1501–1516.

Chavez, R., L. Kemp, and E. Harris. 2004. The social capital health relationship in two disadvantaged neighbourhoods. *Journal of Health Services Research & Policy* 9 (S2): 29–34.

Das, R. 2006. Putting social capital in its place. *Capital & Class* 90: 65–90.

Diani, M., and D. McAdam. 2003. *Social Movements and Networks: Relational Approaches to Collective Action*. Oxford: Oxford University Press.

Edwards, B., and J. D. McCarthy. 2004. Strategy matters: The contingent value of social capital in the survival of local social move organizations. *Social Forces* 83 (2): 621–651.

Edwards, R. 2004. Present and absent in troubling ways: Families and social capital debates. *Sociological Review* 52 (1): 1–21.

Fairclough, N. 2000. *New Labour, New Language?* London: Routledge.

Fine, B. 2001. *Social Capital versus Social Theory: Political Economy and Social Science at the Turn of the Millennium.* London and New York: Routledge.

Foley, M., and B. Edwards. 1998. Beyond Tocqueville: Civil society and social capital in comparative perspective. *American Behavioral Scientist* 42 (1): 5–20.

Fukuyama, F. 1995. Social capital and the global economy. *Foreign Affairs* 74 (5): 89–103.

Giddens, A. 1990. *The Consequences of Modernity.* Cambridge: Polity Press.

Gieryn, T. 1983. Boundary-work and the demarcation of science from non-science. *American Sociological Review* 48: 781–795.

Gomez, M. B., and C. Muntaner. 2005. Urban redevelopment and neighbourhood health in East Baltimore, Maryland: The role of communitarian and institutional social capital. *Critical Public Health* 15 (2): 83–102.

Granovetter, M. S. 1973. The strength of weak ties. *American Journal of Sociology* 78: 1360–1380.

Hawe, P., and A. Shiel. 2000. Social capital and health promotion: A review. *Social Science and Medicine* 51 (6): 871–885.

Jasper, J. M. 1997. *The Art of Moral Protest: Culture, Biography and Creativity in Social Movements.* Chicago: University of Chicago Press.

Jasper, J. M., and J. Poulsen. 1995. Recruiting strangers and friends: Moral shocks and social networks in Animal Rights and Animal Protest. *Social Problems* 42 (4): 493–512.

Kawachi, I., and B. P. Kennedy. 1997. Health and social cohesion: Why care about income inequality. *British Medical Journal* 314: 1037–1040.

Law, A., and W. McNeish. 2007. Contesting the irrational actor model: A case study of mobile phone mast protest. *Sociology* 41 (3): 439–456.

Law, A., and G. Mooney. 2006. The maladies of social capital Critique II: Resisting neo-liberal conformism. *Critique* 34 (3): 253–268.

Leys, C. 2000. *Market-Driven Politics: Neoliberal Democracy and the Public Interest.* London: Verso.

Lochner, K. A., I. Kawachi, R. T. Brennan, and S. L. Buka. 2003. Social capital and neighbourhood mortality rates in Chicago. *Social Science and Medicine* 56 (8): 1797–1805.

Lynch, J., G. Davey-Smith, M. Hillemeier, M. Shaw, T. Raghunathan, and G. Kanlan. 2001. Income inequality, the psychosocial environment and health: Comparisons of wealthy nations. *The Lancet* 358 (9277): 194–200.

Lynch, J. W., P. Due, C. Muntaner, and G. Davey-Smith. 2000. Social capital: Is it a good investment strategy for public health? *Journal of Epidemiology and Community Health* 54 (6): 404–408.

MacKenzie, D. 2001. Mechanizing Proof: Computing, Risk and Trust. Cambridge, Mass: MIT Press.

Marquand, D. 2004. *Decline of the Public: The Hollowing Out of Citizenship.* Cambridge: Polity Press.

Miller, D., and Dinan, W., eds. 2007. *Thinker, Faker, Spinner, Spy: Corporate PR and the Assault on Democracy.* London: Pluto Press.

Milner, H. 2002. *Civic Literacy: How Informed Citizens Make Democracy Work.* Hanover and London: University Press of New England.

Molyneux, M. 2002. Gender and the silences of social capital: Lessons from Latin America. *Development and Change* 33 (2): 167–188.

Morgen, S. 2002. *Into Our Own Hands: The Women's Health Movement in the United States, 1969–1990.* New Brunswick, NJ: Rutgers University Press.

Muntaner, C., J. Lynch, and G. D. Smith. 2001. Social capital, disorganized communities and the Third Way: Understanding the retreat from structural inequalities in epidemiology and public health. *International Journal of Health Services* 31 (2): 213–237.

Navarro, V. 2002. A critique of social capital. *International Journal of Health Services* 32 (3): 423–432.

Olemacher, T. 1996. Bridging people and protest: Social relays of protest groups against low-flying military jets in West Germany. *Social Problems* 43 (2): 197–218.

Paterson, L. 2002. Social capital and constitutional reform. In *New Scotland, New Society: Are Social and Political Ties Fragmenting?,* eds. J. Curtice, D. McCrone, A. Park, and L. Paterson. Edinburgh: Polygon.

Portes, A. 1998. Social capital: Its origins and applications in modern sociology. *Annual Review of Sociology* 24: 1–24.

The Power Inquiry. 2006. *Power to the People: An Independent Inquiry Into Britain's Democracy.* York: Joseph Rowntree Trust [online], [cited . . .]. Available from <http://www.powerinquiry.org>

Putnam, R. D. 1993. *Making Democracy Work: Civic Traditions in Modern Italy.* With R. Leonardi and R.Y. Nanetti. Princeton, N.J: Princeton University Press.

———. 1995. Bowling alone: America's declining social capital. *Journal of Democracy* 6 (1): 812–818.

———. 2000. *Bowling Alone: The Collapse and Revival of American Community.* New York: Simon & Schuster.

———. 2002. Foreword. In *The Role of Social Capital in Development,* eds. C. Grootaert and T. van Bastelaer. New York: Cambridge University Press.

———. 2004. Bowling together. *OECD Observer* March, 242: 14–15.

Scrambler, G., and D. Kelleher 2006. New social and health movements: Issues of representation and change. *Critical Public Health* 16 (3): 219–231.

Sennett, R. 2006. *The Culture of the New Capitalism.* New Haven: Yale University Press.

Stewart, Sir W. 2000. *Mobile Phones and Health.* Didcot: Independent Expert Group on Mobile Phones (IEGMP).

Szreter, S. 1999. A new political economy for New Labour: The importance of social capital. *Renewal* 7 (1): 30–44.

10 The Health Care Outcomes of Trust

A Review of Empirical Evidence

Karen S. Cook and Irena Stepanikova

10.1 INTRODUCTION

This chapter explores how health care access, quality, and related health care outcomes are linked to interpersonal and generalized trust. The types of trust we focus on include trust between patients and physicians, trust or confidence in the medical system and institutions, and trust inherent in patients' networks outside of health care environments. The relationships between these types of trust and health care outcomes are not well understood. Previous research on the antecedents of health care access, utilization, and quality has focused primarily on sociodemographic, neighborhood and geographical characteristics, health insurance, health status, and the type of health care facilities. Andersen (1995) classifies factors that contribute to health care outcomes as (a) enabling factors (e.g., income, type of health care insurance, etc.), (b) need-based factors (e.g., health status, perceived symptoms, etc.), and (c) predisposing factors (e.g., preferences for health care use and other non health-related factors affecting demand for care). Trust, though not explicitly included in Andersen's typology, could be considered a predisposing factor. The decision to seek health care is partially determined by the level of an individual's trust in providers and in medical institutions more broadly. Essentially, a patient who goes to the trouble of visiting a doctor must believe, to some degree, that the health care services she receives will reduce her symptoms, help her heal, and eventually lead to a better quality of life. Several empirical studies provide evidence consistent with the argument that a link exists between trust and health care outcomes. Our goal is to conduct a review of the existing empirical evidence to provide a more comprehensive picture of how various forms of trust relate to health care outcomes and to propose an empirical model of health care outcomes of trust. This model can serve as a base for further empirical research and theoretical development on the topic of trust and health care, as well as a useful tool in the applied realm of policies and interventions intended to improve health care outcomes.

A systematic, empirically grounded approach is needed in light of the proliferating debates about trust. These debates often invoke the concept of social capital including trust as one of its components. As Alex Law outlines in this volume, Putnam (1996), for instance, defines social capital as including networks, norms *and* trust. Social capital has often been depicted as a potential cure-all for a number of society's ills, including poor population health and problems with the health care system. It has also been viewed as helpful in reducing crime, poverty, and economic underdevelopment. Ways to increase social capital in communities and nations have been explored by governmental agencies and research institutions in various countries, as well as by international organizations such as the World Bank.

Yet, the view that social capital is a panacea is unlikely to be accurate, because the concept has often been 'adopted indiscriminately, adapted uncritically, and applied imprecisely' (Woolcock 1998, 197). Among the problems stemming from the imprecise use of this concept, especially when it is used without distinguishing clearly among its components, is the lack of clarity as to exactly which aspects are responsible for the associated social outcomes. Without more precise causal knowledge, it will be difficult to specify the policy implications of the findings. Uncritical use of this concept also limits policy debates. For example, the exclusive focus on building social capital within a community as a mechanism for improving the health of its members may lead policy makers to ignore deep seated causes of health inequalities, including poverty and discrimination. Because of these potential difficulties, more precisely defined *aspects* of social capital need to be examined in a rigorous fashion in relation to specific social outcomes, including better health. We examine empirical evidence on the role of trust in health care access, utilization and quality. We treat trust as a separate dimension of social relations that is clearly related to social capital, rather than as an indicator of social capital per se.

Our interest in how trust relates to health care outcomes arose from an exploratory qualitative study of physician–patient trust (Cook et al. 2004), conducted in 2000 in two clinics in urban Northern California. The study explored how physicians and their patients understood trust and what they perceived to be the effects of managed care on trust between patients and physicians. Linkages between trust and health care quality and access were not among the main foci of this study in the design stage, but they emerged as one of the dominant themes in our focus groups and interviews. Our informants suggested that trust in patient-physician relationships, especially a patient's trust in a physician, develops as a *consequence* of the patient's positive experiences with the availability and quality of health services. Aspects of care that seemed especially important included access to services, technical quality, including physicians' competence to properly diagnose and treat the patient, physicians' communication skills, such as active listening and the ability to deliver information effectively, and socioemotive aspects of care, such as verbal and nonverbal expressions of caring and empathy.

Our data also indicate that the relationship between the quality of health care and trust is reciprocal. Statements to this effect came more often from physicians, who suggested that just as patient trust increases when patients are happy with the quality of the care they receive, the quality of care increases as a consequence of high levels of trust in the patient–physician relationship. High trust facilitates communication, especially about personal or sensitive subjects, such as sexual behavior, drug and alcohol abuse, or mental health. Physicians observed that high-trust patients are more likely to disclose sensitive information that helps them make correct diagnoses and select effective treatments. Physicians reasoned that these patients might get better health outcomes from treatment because they follow recommendations more carefully, and undergo the prescribed procedures even when complicated, costly or uncomfortable.

The exploratory study also revealed the complexity of the concept trust. The various distinct aspects of trust, including patients' trust in individual physicians, physicians' trust in individual patients, patients' trust in physicians in general, and patients' trust in medical institutions, were all relevant in the context of health care delivery. Before examining the empirical research bearing on these relationships, we discuss our conceptual understanding of trust.

10.2   TYPES OF TRUST IN THE CONTEXT OF HEALTH CARE

For the purposes of this study, we treat trust as an *aspect of social relations* that can produce positive social outcomes (although those we trust might not deserve it or might abuse it under some circumstances). Trust is especially important in situations in which one party is more vulnerable than the other or when there is the risk that one party could exploit another. The risk could entail someone failing to fulfill a promise, or it could be much larger as when we trust our health and lives to a physician we presume to be competent and motivated to do what is in our best interest.

The kind of trust that matters most in such situations is *relational trust,* sometimes referred to as interpersonal trust. It can be defined as the trust of one party in another who is perceived to be trustworthy. Individuals assess trustworthiness on the basis of their knowledge of the other party and the assessed commitment of that party to take the truster's interests to heart. According to Hardin (2002), people are motivated to act in a trustworthy manner by their own interest in maintaining a relationship with the truster. Consequently, trust can be understood as 'encapsulated interest' meaning that one party's interests encapsulate the interests of the other party (even if only to maintain the relationship). According to this view, trust is easier to develop in relationships that are mutually valued, because the fear of ending these relationships serves as an incentive to forgo opportunities to betray this trust. Trust is therefore not solely an attribute of an individual (even though people with different personality characteristics and experiences often vary in terms of their capacity for trust) but also of social relations, which are elements of the social networks and social structures in which individuals are embedded (Cook et al. 2005).

The 'encapsulated interest' view of trust is specifically relational and thus appropriate for the study of trust in relationships of various types, in this case between physicians and their patients (or between health care providers, etc.). This general approach is empirically based on the notion that trust is a rare quality that applies to a somewhat limited set of relationships. We almost never trust anyone with respect to everything, thus Hardin's formulation implies that one actor (A) trusts another actor (B) with respect to X (some activity, object or matter at hand). Trust is therefore circumscribed within the relation to particular activities or objects of trust. Although this view has been criticized as limited in the sense that it restricts the scope of trust and does not fit with the colloquial use of the term 'trust' to refer to matters that are not relational, it is clearly more appropriate in empirical studies of trust at the relational level. On the encapsulated interest theory of trust it is quite difficult to conceptualize the trust of one person for a large corporation or institution (as that would not be particular trust or even "relational" in character). It is widely acknowledged that the concept, trust, has many meanings and has been used as a synonym in some contexts for terms like confidence, reliability and trustworthiness. We have attempted to avoid confusion by adopting one specific definition of trust even though we recognize that other investigators have adopted quite different conceptualizations of trust for their purposes.

The most commonly discussed type of relational trust in health care research is *trust of a patient in a physician*. One special characteristic of physician–patient relationships, which distinguishes patient–physician trust from relational trust between more equal parties, such as friends or peers, is the hierarchy between physicians and patients. In hierarchical relationships, one party is typically more powerful. According to Cook et al., 'because individuals in hierarchic relationships are highly motivated to make prudent or intelligent choices when it comes to trust, they monitor a variety of behaviors and the absence of behaviors to determine if they can trust the other person' (2004, 89). Because physicians are usually more powerful than patients, having access to the information and resources patients need, and since the stakes for patients, who entrust their health to their physicians, are commonly high, it is not surprising that patients continuously assess the physician's trustworthiness by monitoring their interactions closely. Patients implicitly and explicitly evaluate the physician's competence and note the physician's communication skills and expressions of caring, which provide further clues about the degree to which the physician is motivated to provide the best possible care (Cook et al. 2004).

Trust of a physician in a patient is another form of relational trust potentially relevant for understanding health care interactions. Even though it is less frequently discussed, several studies suggest that it is a meaningful concept with implications for health care outcomes. Cook et al. (2004) found that physicians use a variety of clues to evaluate their patients' trustworthiness, and sometimes use this information when considering treatment options. Another study (Merrill et al. 2002) showed that physicians treating active drug users fear deception when these patients request prescription drugs. This fear tends to affect how serious the physicians consider complaints about pain to be and, consequently, how they prescribe medication. If a patient has violated trust in the past, the potential for physician mistrust is so great that some physicians insist on written, mutually agreed on contracts outlining 'common expectations as to how the medications will be prescribed and what the consequences will be for aberrant drug-taking behavior' (Olsen and Alford 2006, 115).

Generalized trust is another kind of trust often discussed in the social sciences. It does not reflect evaluation of the trustworthiness of a specific person, but pertains to other persons in general. For Yamagishi and Yamagishi (1994), for example, generalized trust is the 'default' belief in the benign nature of humans, presuming that they can be trusted. The concept of generalized trust poses considerable theoretical and methodological problems. It is difficult to understand precisely what experiences and relationships underpin the responses individuals give to standard generalized trust measures, which typically ask them if they find that most people can be trusted. Simply put, it is unclear who 'most people' in the typical generalized trust question are. What individual respondents understand by 'most people' may vary widely.

To some degree, these difficulties are also present in research considering *a patient's trust in physicians*. Measures of this form of trust typically ask about trust in doctors in general, not in a specific doctor. This more generalized form of trust is particularly important when patients lack other relevant information about a doctor. In such cases, health care interactions may be shaped more by patients' broader ideas of how trustworthy doctors are in general, than by information pertaining to the individual physician with whom the patient interacts. *Trust in health care institutions*, such as hospitals, clinics, health care plans, and health policy actors, is yet another form of generalized trust that may shape health care interactions. According to several authors, trust in institutions is conceptually distinct from trust in a physician and from trust in physicians (Goold and Klipp 2002; Hall et al. 2002; Zheng et al. 2002). It reflects the sense that institutions are reliable and inspire confidence.

10.3   A REVIEW OF THE EMPIRICAL LITERATURE ON TRUST AND HEALTH CARE OUTCOMES

To identify empirical work on the health care outcomes of trust, we searched the PUBMED-MEDLINE, Sociological Abstracts, and PSYCH

INFO online databases.[1] Once we retrieved a relevant study, we examined its references to identify other empirical studies on the topic.

We used the following inclusion criteria to compile the final list of studies:

- The study was published in English in a peer reviewed journal;
- It used an empirical method;
- It made it clear what the object of trust was (i.e., an individual physician, physicians in general, hospitals, etc.);
- It addressed a relationship between trust and one or more health care outcomes, broadly defined and conceived of trust as an antecedent in this relationship. In quantitative studies, trust was treated as an independent variable;
- It found a significant relationship between trust and a health care outcome (if quantitative), or presented evidence for the existence of such a relationship (if qualitative);
- If quantitative analysis was used, potential confounding factors were controlled.

A total of twenty-three studies, published between 1998 and 2006, met the inclusion criteria. They addressed a variety of health care outcomes, ranging from those pertaining to the initial stages of seeking care to symptom improvement and the ability to sustain behavioral changes after visiting a physician. We sorted outcomes into broad categories, including access and utilization, patient communication and involvement in care, services provided by the physician, patient satisfaction, acceptance, compliance, and adherence, ability to perform self-care, behavioral change, early disease detection, and health status. In the following section, we organize the results of our review into subsections by type of trust, addressing first interpersonal trust between an individual patient and a physician and second generalized forms of trust, including trust in physicians and trust in medical institutions.

10.3.1   Interpersonal Trust

Patients' Trust in an Individual Physician

Four studies suggest that patients' trust in a physician is positively related to *health care access and utilization*. Miller, Seib, and Dennie (2001) conducted focus groups with African Americans in a socioeconomically disadvantaged community with a high rate of cardiovascular and other disease. Participants identified issues relevant to accessing and receiving quality health services in their community and ranked these issues in terms of their priority. Issues related to trust ranked high in all focus groups. The participants expressed concerns that doctors lacked comprehensive knowledge and might misdiagnose them or fail to treat them properly. They also feared that physicians might deny them the newest medicines for insurance reasons. Lack of trust due to negative encounters with providers was especially important among youth, who rated mistrust of their health care providers as the most important psychosocial barrier to accessing care. Additional evidence that mistrust can hinder access to care among some groups comes from a study of reported barriers to health services among American Indians and non-Hispanic whites in a probability sample of Minnesota health care program enrollees (Call et al. 2006). Mistrust of their child's provider was one barrier to obtaining health care reported more commonly by American Indian parents than by white parents.

Two quantitative studies considered trust and health care utilization. One of them (Mollborn, Stepanikova, and Cook 2005) used a representative cross-sectional sample of Americans to examine the relationships between unmet health care needs and patients' trust in a physician, measured by a 4-item scale. In multivariate models controlling for sociodemographic factors, health status, health insurance, and satisfaction with choice of physician, the likelihood of reporting unmet health care needs and delayed care was negatively related to patients' trust in a physician in most patient groups. However, for Blacks, Hispanics, the poor, and the uninsured, no relationship between trust in a physician and delayed care was found. The authors suggest that among these disadvantaged patients, considering trust when making decisions about health care is a luxury they cannot afford, since their health care decisions are constrained by more pressing factors such as financial concerns, availability of child care and transportation, or the ability to choose their health care provider. Ling, Klein, and Dang (2006) studied the relationship between trust in information from a health care provider and utilization of preventive services. In a national probability sample of 2,670 respondents greater than 50 years of age, the use of colorectal cancer screening tests was positively related to trust in cancer information obtained from a health care provider.

Patient–physician communication as an outcome associated with patients' trust in a physician was reported in two studies. Bell et al. (2001) examined unvoiced patients' desires during physician visits, using data from 909 patients visiting family practitioners, internal medicine specialists, and cardiologists. They also measured trust in a physician, using a 9-item scale. Patients with higher pre-visit trust were more likely to communicate their desires during visits. A qualitative study by Rhodes and Hergenrather (2002) indicated that men who had sex with men were more inclined to communicate information about their risky behavior to their physicians if they trusted that physicians would not judge them. Some reported that they did not talk to their physicians because they did not trust that the physician would be comfortable discussing their sexual orientation. One participant, for instance, said, "I might tell him . . . if only he was relaxed, and I knew

I could trust him to respond without reaction" (133). Finally, communicative behaviors indicating *involvement in care,* as evidenced by patients' requests for services, were addressed by Thom et al. (2002), who reported that after controlling for physicians' and patients' sociodemographic characteristics and characteristics of care, patients' pre-visit trust in a physician was positively related to requests for medical information and new medications during visits.

The same study found that pre-visit trust in a physician was associated with reports of *services provided by the physician,* measured after the visit. Patients with lower levels of trust were more likely to report that they requested medical information, examination, diagnostic service, new medication, or a referral but the physician did not provide the services. Another study investigates the perceived fulfillment of patient requests, an outcome closely related to services provided by the physician (Kravitz et al. 2002). Patients visiting family practitioners, internal medicine specialists and cardiologists rated trust in the treating physician before the visit. After the visit, they reported requests for services they made and the physician's responses to these requests. Fulfillment of requests for services was significantly lower among patients who reported lower trust in their physician.

Patients' *satisfaction* was addressed in five studies. In a cross-sectional study of 7204 adults employed by the Commonwealth of Massachusetts, patients' trust in a physician, measured by a subscale of the Primary Care Assessment Survey (PCAS), was positively related to satisfaction with a primary care physician (Safran et al. 1998). In a survey of 414 patients in twenty family practices, patients' trust in a physician, measured by an 11-item Trust in Physician Scale (TPS), predicted higher levels of patient satisfaction with several areas of care provided by their physician, measured six months later (Thom et al. 1999). Thom et al. (2002) administered a survey to 732 patients in two managed care settings. They found that patients' pre-visit trust in a physician, measured by TPS, was positively associated with patients' satisfaction with the services provided, measured immediately after the visit and two weeks later. Using data from a cross-sectional telephone survey, Keating et al. (2002) reported a positive relationship between patients' trust in a physician and satisfaction with care. This relationship was also suggested by Baker et al. (2003), who asked patients in the United States (N=418) and United Kingdom (N=650) to complete a pre-visit questionnaire about trust in a regular doctor and a post-visit questionnaire about satisfaction with the visit. Pre-visit trust in a regular physician was strongly associated with post-visit satisfaction, especially among patients who visited their regular doctor. *Unmet patients' expectations,* an outcome closely related to low satisfaction, was examined by Bell et al. (2002). Pre-visit trust, measured by a 9-item scale, was negatively associated with the likelihood of reporting at least one unmet expectation after the visit. Unmet expectations pertained to clinical data collection (e.g., failure to prepare for a visit), allocation of clinical resources (e.g., tests, medications, referrals), providing information and counseling, and other matters.

Seven studies dealt with relationships between patients' trust in a physician and *acceptance, compliance, and adherence* to therapeutic regimens. Thom et al. (1999) found that trust in a physician was positively related to patients' reports six months later that they always take most or all of their prescribed medications. Safran et al. (1998) reported that patients' trust in a physician was positively related to patients' reports of adherence to physician advice about smoking, alcohol use, seat belt use, diet, exercise, stress, and safe sex practices. In a cross-sectional survey of 205 HIV-infected prisoners eligible for antiretroviral therapy, higher levels of trust in a physician, measured by TPS, were related to a higher likelihood of accepting antiretroviral therapy (Altice, Mostashari, and Friedland 2001). Roberts (2002) conducted in-depth interviews with 28 HIV-positive patients to explore factors influencing adherence to antiretroviral medication. One basic theme emerging from the data was 'If you don't trust your doctor, you won't trust (and take) your meds' (47). For some patients, trusting their physician and seeing that the physician believes in antiretroviral medications helped them adhere to this regimen.

Another qualitative study explored factors influencing willingness to undergo invasive cardiac testing among candidates for this procedure (Collins et al. 2002). Focus groups with thirteen patients and transcripts of patients' discussions with their health providers revealed that trust in a provider influenced candidates' comfort and preferences regarding cardiac testing. Trust seemed especially important for Black patients, who consistently expressed preference for building a trusting relationship with physicians before agreeing to invasive testing. In another study, Keating et al. (2002) found that patients with higher levels of trust in a physician at the time of a visit were more likely to report that they intended to follow their physicians' advice when interviewed two weeks after the visit. Similarly, Thom et al. (2002) showed that patients with higher levels of pre-visit trust in a physician were more likely to indicate two weeks after the visit that they strongly intended to adhere to the physician's advice. Finally, a study using a cross-sectional survey with 912 diabetes patients recruited from five Veterans Administration health systems (Piette et al. 2005) examined adherence to prescription medication among, patients' trust in a physician, measured by a standard scale, moderated the effects of cost-related constraints and pressures on prescription medication underuse. Patients with higher out-of-pocket costs were more likely to forgo medications when their trust in a physician was low. Among low-trust patients, but not among high-trust patients, low income was associated with underuse of medication. Mainous et al. (2001) reported a relationship between trust and *early disease detection*. Using data from cross-sectional face-to-face interviews with 119 newly diagnosed breast and colorectal cancer patients, they found that trust in one's primary care physician was related to detecting cancer at an earlier stage.

Self-reported *health status* was linked to trust in three studies. In a study described earlier, trust in a physician, measured by a subset of the PCAS, was positively associated with perceived changes in general health status compared to four years ago (Safran et al. 1998). Keating et al. (2002) found that two weeks after a visit, patients with higher levels of trust measured at the time of the visit were more likely to report their symptoms had improved. Symptom improvement was also examined by Thom et al. (2002). Two weeks after a visit to a physician, patients rated their symptoms on a scale ranging from 'much worse' to 'much better.' Their ratings were positively associated with trust in a physician, measured before the visit.

Physicians' Trust in a Patient

One qualitative study using interviews and observations of physician–patient interactions in an urban public hospital demonstrated how physicians' mistrust of patients can affect their medical decisions about prescribing medications (Merrill et al. 2002). Physicians treating patients who were active drug users feared their patients would try to deceive them to obtain drugs. Physicians lacked consistent criteria to judge patients' complaints, especially as they concerned pain and prescribing opiates, and avoided engaging patients' key complaints, thus ignoring important information.

10.3.2 Generalized Forms of Trust in Health Care Providers and Medical Institutions

Trust in Physicians

Bonds et al. (2004) conducted a cross-sectional survey of 320 medically underserved diabetes patients in rural North Carolina. They measured patients' trust in physicians at the clinic using five items from the Wake Forest University Trust Scale, such as "All in all, you trust the doctors at 'this clinic' completely." Trust in physicians was positively associated with global assessments of the overall *ability to perform self-care* for diabetes and negatively associated with perceived difficulty of exercising regularly, checking blood sugar, and checking feet for sores. Trust was also negatively associated with perceived hassles associated with diabetes self-care tasks, such as remembering to take medication and test blood sugar, making meal plans, avoiding particular foods, and organizing daily routines around medical care.

Rutten et al. (2005) studied patients' trust in advice from health care providers. For the purposes of this review, we consider it an aspect of trust in health care providers. In a cross-sectional survey of a sample representative of the American population, respondents rated how much they trusted information from health care providers. People who had smoked regularly at some point in their lives, but had now abstained from smoking for a year or more, had higher levels of trust in advice from health care providers compared to current smokers. This study suggests that trust in advice from providers is related to *the ability to sustain a desirable behavioral change.*

Trust in Medical Institutions

Nicholson et al. (2006) reported a cross-sectional study linking trust in the medical community to *utilization of care.* Among 131 adult primary care patients with moderately to severely disabling migraines, mistrust in the medical community, measured by the 11-item Medical Mistrust Scale, was negatively related to the likelihood of seeing a doctor for migraines. Patients with higher medical mistrust were also less likely to get a prescription for migraine medication, which suggests a relationship between trust in medical institutions and *obtaining health services.* LaVeist, Nickerson and Bowie (2000) conducted a cross-sectional survey of 1784 cardiac patients discharged from a hospital. Mistrust in hospitals, measured by an index of items such as 'Patients have sometimes been deceived or misled at hospitals' was negatively related to patient *satisfaction* with several aspects of care received from the main doctor during hospitalization.

Balkrishnan et al. (2004) conducted a longitudinal study of enrollees in a health maintenance organization (HMO)[2] in the southwestern United States. To reduce costs, many HMOs encourage their enrollees to seek care from a primary care physician within their provider network, rather than seeing specialists or outside-of-network physicians. Balkrishnan et al. were interested in whether HMO enrollees who trust their insurer were more likely to seek their care from a primary care provider within their network rather than seeing a specialist or another physician who is not a part of this network. They found that this was in fact the case. Trust in managed care insurers, measured at the baseline, was positively associated with *seeking care from a primary care provider,* as opposed to seeking care from another doctor.

Trust in government-sponsored health care emerged as one factor contributing to *accepting hepatitis B vaccination* in a qualitative study of men who have sex with men (Rhodes and Hergenrather 2002). This study explored how these men perceive barriers to vaccination. Distrust of government-sponsored health care was one perceived barrier, especially prominent among African American participants, who often referred to the Tuskegee syphilis study[3] to explain their fear of government-supported health care. These participants feared vaccination might be a scientific experiment designed to make them sick.

10.4 A MODEL OF THE RELATIONSHIPS BETWEEN
TRUST AND VARIOUS HEALTH CARE OUTCOMES

The studies included in our review provide considerable evidence that several forms of trust have implications for health care outcomes. Based on this evidence, we propose a model of the health care outcomes of trust, illustrated in Figure 1. Depicted in boldly outlined rectangles are the three

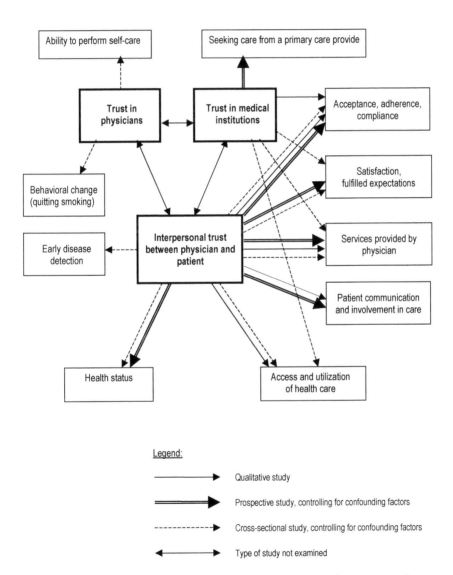

Figure 10.1. A Model of the Health Care Outcomes of Trust Based on a Review of the Empirical

forms of trust indicated by our review to influence health care outcomes. They are interpersonal trust between physicians and patients, trust in physicians, and trust in medical institutions. Notably, since our review yielded no studies of generalized trust in people *outside of health care environments,* this form of trust does not appear in the model.

Interpersonal trust between physicians and patients, depicted at the center of Figure 1, includes patients' trust in a physician as well physicians' trust in a patient. Our review primarily yielded studies of patients' trust in a physician. Physicians' trust in a patient was addressed only by a single study reported by Merrill et al. (2002). This study stressed the reciprocal character of interpersonal trust between physicians and patients. This conclusion is consistent with the findings of our exploratory study (Cook et al. 2004), as well as with other work on trust in health care settings (Thorne and Robinson 1988). The evidence supports the strategy of considering interpersonal trust between physicians and patients as a meaningful category, encompassing patient's trust in a physician, physicians' trust in their patients and the mutual influence of these two aspects of trust.

Trust in physicians in Figure 1 is one form of generalized trust in health care providers that is relevant in health care settings. In the studies we reviewed, it was represented by trust in doctors at a particular clinic and trust in advice from providers. Another form of trust shown in Figure 1 is trust in medical institutions. This category encompasses trust in the healthcare system, trust in the medical community, trust in insurers, trust in managed care, and trust in government-sponsored health care.

We included studies of mistrust together with studies of trust in our model. The studies we reviewed addressed mistrust in a health care provider (Miller, Seib, and Dennie 2001; Call et al. 2006), physicians' mistrust of patients (Merrill et al. 2002), mistrust in the medical community (Nicholson et al. 2006), and mistrust in hospitals (LaVeist, Nickerson, and Bowie 2000). Some scholars have argued that mistrust is conceptually distinct from low levels of trust (Cook et al. 2004). If such an argument is correct, combining mistrust with trust may be problematic. Yet, other studies suggest that mistrust behaves similarly to low trust in relation to the health care outcomes of interest to us. Mistrust relates negatively to health care access and utilization (Miller, Seib, and Dennie 2001; Call et al. 2006), which we would expect based on studies showing that these outcomes decrease among patients with lower levels of trust (Mollborn, Stepanikova, and Cook 2005; Ling, Klein and Dang. 2006). Similarly, patients with lower levels of institutional trust have lower levels of satisfaction (Gordon et al. 2006)[4], which is what LaViest et al.'s (2000) study of institutional mistrust would lead us to expect if mistrust behaves similarly to low trust in relation to satisfaction. Based on these similarities, we find it justifiable, for the purpose of our model, to place studies addressing mistrust in the same category as studies addressing trust in the same object (e.g., mistrust in a physician is grouped together with trust in a physician), even though we leave open the possibility that mistrust is conceptually distinct from trust.

Before discussing how the three forms of trust relate to health care outcomes, we briefly address the relationships among them. These relationships were not part of our empirical review but other evidence indicates their interconnectedness. Zheng et al. (2002), for instance, found that trust in an individual physician was positively related to trust in insurers. Dugan, Trachtenberg and Hall (2005) reported that trust in a physician positively correlated both with trust in an insurer and trust in the medical profession. Bonds et al. (2004) showed an association between trust in a primary care provider and trust in doctors and nurses at the hospital. A relationship between general trust in physicians and trust in an individual physician was also reported by Hall et al. (2002). In Figure 1, the relationships among the three aspects of trust are depicted by the double-sided arrows. We use these types of arrows to indicate that empirical studies reported a relationship, but that in this project, we did not analyze specifically what types of methodologies (i.e. qualitative, cross-sectional, prospective, etc.) these empirical studies used.

The part of the model directly derived from our empirical review pertains to relationships between the three forms of trust and various health care outcomes. To better understand what type of evidence supports each specific part of our model, we use three types of arrows to depict relationships between trust and health care outcomes in Figure 1. Distinguishing between the types of studies is important, as the method used in each study determines the conclusions that can be drawn, especially as they pertain to causality. Each arrow indicates one *type* of evidence supporting a particular relationship (not the number of studies using this evidence). Simple arrows represent qualitative evidence, which helps us understand mechanisms connecting variables, especially as perceived by informants. Because qualitative studies typically use small convenience samples, conclusions are stronger if also supported by other more representative studies. Quantitative studies using cross-sectional methodology, represented by dashed arrows in Figure 1, can more accurately describe larger populations but are not authoritative sources of information on causality. We limited our attention to cross-sectional studies using statistical controls that isolate potential confounding factors. Finally, prospective studies that include data collected over time are represented by double arrows. They are most suitable among the three types of evidence for drawing causal inferences. Again, we included only those prospective studies that applied statistical controls. This strategy increases the likelihood that the relationships found are, in fact, causal, but it cannot guard against omitted factors that can make causal conclusions erroneous. None of the studies reviewed in this chapter presents clear evidence that a relationship is causal or that it flows in a particular direction, but some studies provide stronger evidence than others suggesting that causal relationships *may* exist.

Even a perfunctory review of Figure 1 reveals that evidence on interpersonal trust between a physician and a patient is more comprehensive and varied compared to evidence on generalized forms of trust in health care providers and medical institutions. Interpersonal trust is connected to most outcome categories and is addressed more commonly by prospective studies, which yield evidence generally considered suggestive of causality. Evidence is especially strong for linkages between interpersonal trust and services provided by a physician and patients' communication, satisfaction, adherence, and health status. Each of these linkages is supported by two or more types of empirical evidence, one of which is prospective. Institutional trust is related to a respectable number of outcome categories in Figure 1, but the evidence for these relationships is mainly cross-sectional, making it less clear whether aspects of health care linked to institutional trust are its consequences or its antecedents. Clearly, the smallest number of studies considers general trust in physicians. This may be a result of the fact that interpersonal trust has commanded the attention of health care researchers for a longer time than generalized forms of trust in health care providers and medical institutions. As research progresses in the future, we will see whether the relative paucity of evidence on health care outcomes of generalized forms of trust in health care providers and medical institutions, revealed by our review, is an artifact of a research niche that is still immature or whether it reflects a true lack of significant relationships between these forms of trust and health care outcomes.

10.5 POTENTIAL MECHANISMS LINKING TRUST TO HEALTH CARE OUTCOMES

Why do the relationships exist between trust and health care outcomes, as shown in our model? What are the mechanisms connecting trust to its outcomes? Our review did not address these questions, focusing instead strictly on empirical evidence for *the existence* of these relationships. Yet, theoretical scholarship on trust in the health care context offers some preliminary insights, which we briefly consider in this section, before discussing some of the limitations of our review.

Common to recent research is the emphasis on trust as an aspect of social networks that enable people to *access information and use it efficiently*. For decades, social scientists have known that social networks play a crucial role in transmitting information. More recently, this knowledge has been fruitfully applied to health care topics. Kawachi and Berkman (2000), for example, argue that networks are the primary channels through which information travels and can aid the dissemination of knowledge about health and health care, including information about providers, insurance, treatment, preventive care, and ways to gain access. Networks are especially useful if they include individuals with specialized knowledge (e.g., social workers) or community organizations that provide such knowledge. Higher levels of interpersonal trust among residents of a community may result in quicker diffusion and uptake of this knowledge.

Arthur (2002) demonstrates in the case of kidney transplants how networks provide information that enables people to make complex medical decisions. She argues that 'patients . . . who receive information about the transplantation referral and evaluation procedures from contacts and other weak ties in their social network are more likely to pursue such a procedure.' She discusses how disadvantaged social groups, particularly African Americans, lack these useful networks and consequently have lower acceptance of transplantation.

From Arthur's example, it is easy to see how trust would be an important factor in making use of health care information, should it become available through social networks, and how such information may eventually lead to changes in health status. To seriously consider transplantation, one would have to trust the source of the information about its benefits. If such information came from a trusted source, a potential candidate for the procedure may find the information credible, consider it, and eventually take steps toward getting a transplant, which, if successful, would result in improved health status. If, however, the very same information came from a distrusted source, the candidate may not even pay attention to it. She may forgo the potentially beneficial procedure and her health may deteriorate.

Similarly, Thiede (2005) argues that trust is an important factor in exchanges of information. Since most interactions between patients and health care providers involve information exchange, trust can aid in making these exchanges effective. A successful exchange of information can improve access to health care, defined as the freedom to use health care, or, more precisely, the 'individual ability to give direction to one's will to use health care services' (1453) that already exist in the individual's opportunity structure.

Another explanation concerns *cooperative behavior,* which, based on experimental evidence, increases as interpersonal trust increases (Cook and Cooper 2003). More cooperation between physicians and patients can help accomplish tasks needed to diagnose and treat the patient more efficiently. A related explanation is that trust potentially lowers *transaction costs.* According to Thom (2001), transaction costs lowered in trusting physician–patient relationships include 'those incurred by a need to reassure patients (e.g., ordering additional tests and referrals) or by inefficiencies due to incomplete disclosure of information by the patient.'

Another potential mechanism linking trust to better health care outcomes is the idea that trust motivates the parties involved to behave in trustworthy ways. One partner's trust breeds *trustworthiness* of the other partner, which, in turn, fosters mutual trust. In the context of health care, this mechanism may motivate physicians who treat high-trust patients to provide better services. In fact, patients' trust may be the most important motivator for physicians when other effective accountability mechanisms are missing. As the World Bank (2006) explains, 'in some remote rural areas, it is difficult and costly for government agencies to check up on health workers to ensure that they are at their posts, providing quality care. Sometimes, the relationship that the provider has with the community is the primary incentive for working hard.' In a similar way, a patient who knows that her physician trusts her may be more motivated to behave in ways that honor this trust by disclosing sensitive health-related information and complying with the physician's advice and adhering to the recommended medical regimens, even if onerous.

An explanation involving motivation has also been proposed to explain the link between institutional trust and health care access. Mollborn et al. (2005) argued that trust in the health care system motivated people to make use of the system by selecting a usual source of care and then seeking care at that source. People who do not use the health care system may not do so partially because of systemic mistrust, possibly generated by negative experiences with the quality of care received in the past.

10.6   LIMITATIONS AND CONCLUSIONS

In recent years, research on trust and health has proliferated. The published works vary widely in their quality and approaches. They range from opinion essays to theoretical pieces, policy recommendations, and empirical studies, making it difficult to keep up with this growing literature without devoting considerable time and effort to reading original sources. In particular, it has become increasingly difficult to distinguish which of the claims about linkages between trust and health outcomes that appear in literature are supported by empirical findings and which are more speculative in nature. Therefore, it is important to provide careful reviews of existing empirical research that will enable researchers to quickly gain orientation in the growing literature. A limitation of the existing research and our model, however, is that the evidence supporting the proposed model consists solely of patients' reports. More objective studies of health care outcomes are rare, possibly because the collection of objective data tends to be costly and time-consuming. For some health care outcomes, such as satisfaction and adherence to physician advice about some risk behaviors, objective measurement is impractical or impossible. Given these difficulties, it is not surprising that our review produced no studies using objective measures of health care outcomes. Therefore, it appears prudent to keep in mind that the health care outcomes considered in our model represent *patients' perceptions* of these outcomes. Patients' perceptions are important, as they reveal a great deal about patients' experiences with care. Yet, they may not relate to trust in the same way as more objectively measured aspects of health and health care. It is easy to see how patients' trust may correlate more strongly with self-reported health than with measures of health status derived from medical records. Future research is needed to better understand how these two types of measures relate to trust.

Another limitation is that our review did not consider studies of factors contributing to various forms of trust in health care settings. Such studies were beyond the scope of this review, but they help us understand the complex relationships between trust and aspects of health care. Some of these studies address how physicians' behavior influences patient trust in a physician (Goold and Klipp 2002) and trust in medical institutions (e.g., Berrios-Rivera et al. 2006). Although these studies conceive of trust as an outcome of physician behaviors, the possibility that some of these behaviors are, in fact, outcomes of trust remains open. The possibility that the direction of causality between physician behavior and patient–physician trust is reciprocal seems especially likely if we consider the relationship between physicians and patients to be inherently reciprocal. Future research should address these and the related issues we have discussed to determine more precisely the extent to which the types of trust we have identified in our empirical review matter for improving health care and health outcomes as well as the point at which they become relevant.

NOTES

1. We searched for abstracts that contained the term "trust" together with "health care quality," "quality of health care," "health care access," "access to health care," "health care use," "health care utilization," "utilization of health care," "health care underuse," or "health care overuse."
2. HMOs are organizations in the United States that act both as health insurers and health care providers. They cover specified medical services delivered by designated in-network providers.
3. Tuskegee Study of Untreated Syphilis in the Negro Male (1932–1972) was conducted by the U.S. Public Health Service with 399 infected and 201 uninfected African American men residing in Macon County, Alabama, to examine the course of untreated syphilis. The subjects were not told that they had syphilis and were denied penicillin treatment. The study is a prominent example of unethical medical research and racism in medicine.
4. Gordon et al.'s (2006) study did not meet the inclusion criteria as it modeled trust as an outcome of satisfaction.

REFERENCES

Altice, F. L., F. Mostashari, and G. H. Friedland. 2001. Trust and the acceptance of and adherence to antiretroviral therapy. *Journal of Acquired Immune Deficiency Syndrome* 28 (1): 47–58.
Andersen, R. M. 1968. A behavioral model of families' use of health services. *Research Series No. 15.* Center for Health Administration Studies, University of Chicago.
Andersen, R. M. 1995. Revisiting the Behavioural Model and Accesss to Medical Care: Does it Matter? *Journal of Health and Social Behaviour* 36:1–10.
Arthur, T. 2002. The role of social networks: A novel hypothesis to explain the phenomenon of racial disparity in kidney transplantation. *American Journal of Kidney Disorder* 40 (4): 678–681.
Baker, R. 2002. Exploration of the relationship between continuity, trust in regular doctors and patient satisfaction with consultations with family doctors. *Scandinavian Journal of Primary Health Care* 21 (1): 27–32.
Balkrishnan, R., M. A. Hall, S. Blackwelder, and D. Bradley. 2004. Trust in insurers and access to physicians: Associated enrollee behaviors and changes over time. *BMC Health Services Research* 39 (4-1): 813–824.

Bell, R. A., R. L. Kravitz, D. Thom, E. Krupat, and R. Azari. 2001. Unsaid but not forgotten: Patients' unvoiced desires in office visits. *Archives of Internal Medicine* 161 (16): 1977–1984.
———. 2002. Unmet expectations for care and the patient–physician relationship. *Journal of General Internal Medicine* 17 (11): 817–824.
Berrios-Rivera, J. P., R. L. Street Jr., M. G. Garcia Popa-Lisseanu, M. A. Kallen, M. N. Richardson, N. M. Janssen, D. M. Marcus, J. D. Reveille, N. B. Warner, and M. E. Suarez-Almazor. 2006. Trust in physicians and elements of the medical interaction in patients with rheumatoid arthritis and systemic lupus erythematosus. *Arthritis and Rheumatism* 55 (3): 385–393.
Bonds, D. E., Foley, K. L., Dugan, E., Hall, M. A., Extrom, P. 2004. An exploration of patients' trust in physicians in training. *Journal of Health Care for the Poor and Underserved* 15 (2): 294–306.
Call, K. T., D. D. McAlpine, P. J. Johnson, T. J. Beebe, J. A. McRae, and Y. Song. 2006. Barriers to care among American Indians in public health care programs. *Medical Care* 44 (6): 595–600.
Collins, T. C., J. A. Clark, L. A. Petersen, and N. R. Kressin. 2002. Racial differences in how patients perceive physician communication regarding cardiac testing. *Medical Care* 40 (1 Suppl): 27–34.
Cook, K. S., and R. Cooper. 2003. Experimental studies of cooperation, trust, and social exchange. In *Trust, Reciprocity and Gains from Association: Interdisciplinary Lessons from Experimental Research*. New York, NY: Russell Sage Foundation.
Cook, K. S., R. Kramer, D. Thom, I. Stepanikova, S. B. Mollborn, and R. Cooper. 2004. Trust and distrust in patient–physician relationships: Perceived determinants of high and low trust relationships in managed care settings. In *Trust and Distrust across Organizational Contexts,* eds. R. Kramer and K. S. Cook. New York, NY: Russell Sage.
Cook, K., Hardin, R., Levi, M. 2005. *Cooperation without trust?* New York: Russell Sage Publications.
Dugan, E., F. Trachtenberg, and M. A Hall. 2005. Development of abbreviated measures to assess patient trust in a physician, a health insurer, and the medical profession. *BMC Health Services Research* 5: 64.
Goold, S. D., and G. Klipp. 2002. Managed care members talk about trust. *Social Science Medicine* 54 (6): 879-888.
Gordon, H. S., R. L. Street, Jr., B. F. Sharf, P. A. Kelly, and J. Souchek. 2006. Racial differences in trust and lung cancer patients' perceptions of physician communication. *Journal of Clinical Oncology* 24 (6): 904–909.
Hall, M. A., F. Camacho, E. Dugan, and R. Balkrishnan. 2002. Trust in the medical profession: Conceptual and measurement issues. *BMC Health Services Research* 37 (5): 1419–1439.
Hardin, R. 2002. *Trust and Trustworthiness.* New York, NY: Russell Sage Foundation.
Kawachi, I., and L. F. Berkman. 2000. Social cohesion, social capital, and health. In *Social Epidemiology,* eds. I. Kawachi and L. F.Berkman. New York, NY: Oxford University Press.
Keating, N. L., D. C. Green, A. C. Kao, J. A. Gazmararian, V. Y. Wu, and P. D. Cleary. 2002. How are patients' specific ambulatory care experiences related to trust, satisfaction, and considering changing physicians? *Journal of General Internal Medicine* 17 (1): 29–39.
Kravitz, R. L., R. A. Bell, R. Azari, E. Krupat, S. Kelly-Reif, and D. Thom. 2002. Request fulfillment in office practice: Antecedents and relationship to outcomes. *Medical Care* 40 (1): 38–51.

LaVeist, T. A., K. J. Nickerson, and J. V. Bowie. 2000. Attitudes about racism, medical mistrust, and satisfaction with care among African American and white cardiac patients. *Medical Care Research and Review* 57 Suppl 1: 146–161.

Ling, B. S., W. M. Klein, and Q. Dang. 2006. Relationship of communication and information measures to colorectal cancer screening utilization: Results from HINTS. *Journal of Health Communication* 11 (Suppl.): 181–190.

Mainous, Arch G. III, R. Baker, M. M. Love, D. Pereira Gray, and J. M. Gill. 2001. Continuity of care and trust in one's physician: Evidence from primary care in the United States and the United Kingdom. *Family Medicine* 33: 22–27.

Merrill, J. O., L. A. Rhodes, R. A. Deyo, G. A. Marlatt, and K. A. Bradley. 2002. Mutual mistrust in the medical care of drug users: The keys to the "narc" cabinet. *Journal of General Internal Medicine* 17 (5): 327–333.

Miller, S. T., H. M. Seib, and S. P. Dennie. 2001. African American perspectives on health care: The voice of the community. *The Journal of Ambulatory Care Management* 24 (3): 37–44.

Mollborn, S., I. Stepanikova, and K. S. Cook. 2005. Delayed care and unmet needs among health care system users: When does fiduciary trust in a physician matter? *BMC Health Services Research* 40 (6 Pt 1): 1898–1917.

Nicholson, R. A., M. Rooney, K. Vo, E. O'Laughlin, and M. Gordon. 2006. Migraine care among different ethnicities: Do disparities exist? *Headache* 46 (5): 754–765.

Olsen, Y., and D. P. Alford. 2006. Chronic pain management in patients with substance use disorders. *Advanced Studies in Medicine* 6 (3): 111–123.

Piette, J. D., M. Heisler, S. Krein, and E. A. Kerr. 2005. The role of patient–physician trust in moderating medication nonadherence due to cost pressures. *Archives of Internal Medicine* 165 (15): 1749–1755.

Putnam, R. D. 1996. The strange disappearance of civic America. *The American Prospect* 24: 34–48.

Rhodes, S. D., and K. C. Hergenrather. 2002. Exploring hepatitis B vaccination acceptance among young men who have sex with men: Facilitators and barriers. *Preventive Medicine* 35 (2): 128–134.

Roberts, K. J. 2002. Physician–patient relationships, patient satisfaction, and antiretroviral medication adherence among HIV-infected adults attending a public health clinic. *AIDS Patient Care and STDs* 16 (1): 43–50.

Rutten, L., J. Finney, K. Wanke, and E. Augustson. 2005. Systems and individual factors associated with smoking status: Evidence from HINTS. *American Journal of Health Behaviour* 29 (4): 302–310.

Safran, D. G., D. A. Taira, W. H. Rogers, M. Kosinski, J. E. Ware, and A. R. Tarlov. 1998. Linking primary care performance to outcomes of care. *Journal of Family Practice* 47: 213–220.

Thiede, M. 2005. Information and access to health care: Is there a role for trust? *Social Science Medicine* 61 (7): 1452–1462.

Thom, D. H. 2001. Physician behaviors that predict patient trust. *Journal of Family Practice* 50 (4): 323–328.

Thom, D. H., R. L. Kravitz, R. A. Bell, E. Krupat, and R. Azari. 2002. Patient trust in the physician: Relationship to patient requests. *Family Practice* 19 (5): 476–483.

Thom, D. H., K. M. Ribisl, A. L. Stewart, and D. A. Luke. 1999. Further validation of a measure of patients' trust in their physician: The Trust in Physician Scale. *Medical Care* 37: 510–517.

Thorne, S. E., and C. A. Robinson. 1988. Reciprocal trust in health care relationships. *Journal of Advanced Nursing* 13 (6): 782–789.

Woolcock, M. 1998. Social capital and economic development: A critical review. *Theory and Society* 27 (2):151–208.

World Bank. 2006. Social Capital for Development [online], Available from <http://www1.worldbank.org/prem/poverty/scapital/index.htm>

Yamagishi, T., and M. Yamagishi. 1994. Trust and commitment in the United States and Japan. *Motivation and Emotion* 18: 129–166.

Zheng, B., M. A. Hall, E. Dugan, K. E. Kidd, and D. Levine. 2002. Development of a scale to measure patients' trust in health insurers. *BMC Health Services Research* 37 (1): 187–202.

Contributors

Julie Brownlie is a Sociology Lecturer at the University of Stirling. Her research and teaching interests include social theory, sociology of childhood, the body and trust. She has been researching trust in relation to childhood and health for several years and is currently exploring trust in the context of an ESRC funded research study on emotional support and talk.

Karen S. Cook is the Ray Lyman Wilbur Professor of Sociology, Chair of the Department of Sociology and Director of the Institute for Research in the Social Sciences (IRiSS) at Stanford University. She is a member of the American Academy of Arts and Sciences and the National Academy of Sciences. In 2004 she received the Cooley-Mead award for career contributions to social psychology from the American Sociological Association. Her research interests include social exchange relations, power dynamics, negotiation, trust, physician–patient relations, and social networks. Her most recent book is *Cooperation without Trust?* (2005), published by the Russell Sage Foundation (co-authored with R. Hardin and M. Levi).

Sarah Cunningham-Burley is Professor of Medical and Family Sociology at the University of Edinburgh. She is based in the Division of Community Health Sciences (Public Health Sciences section) within the College of Medicine and Veterinary Medicine and also at the Centre for Research on Families and Relationships (CRFR), where she is a codirector. Her research interests include sociological aspects of genetics and health; public engagement in science; young people, children and health; families, relationships and health.

Joyce Davidson is Assistant Professor of Geography, cross-appointed to Women's Studies, at Queen's University, Kingston, Ontario. Following her UK-based doctoral research on agoraphobia, which formed the basis of *Phobic Geographies: The Phenomenology and Spatiality of Identity* (Ashgate, 2003), she developed a research and teaching programme focused around gendered experience of embodiment and emotional health. She has published in a range of journals across various disciplines, including *Body and Society, Hypatia,* and *Social Science and Medicine,* is coauthor of *Subjectivities, Knowledges and Feminist Geographies* (Rowman and Littlefield, 2002), and coeditor of *Emotional Geographies* (Ashgate, 2005).

Alexandra Greene is a Senior Research Fellow in the Health Services Research Unit, at the University of Aberdeen. She leads the Health Care Users theme in the Delivery of Care Programme, which conducts research on the social and cultural contexts of health and illness and, in particular, ways to involve service users (particularly the young) in research and development agenda setting in the NHS. As part of her interest in interdisciplinary dialogue, she cofounded the Nexus Programme, an interdisciplinary research forum for social scientists, health professionals and patients, and is a member of DAWN, an international initiative to support Youth Ambassadors for diabetes.

Stephen Greene qualified from University College Hospital Medical School, London and then pursued a career in Child Health with positions in Oxford, Great Ormond Street, London, the Kinderspital Hospital, Zurich and Guy's Hospital, London. He was appointed a Consultant Paediatric Endocrinologist for Tayside in 1987 and Reader in Child and Adolescent Health, University of Dundee, in 2001. He has a specific research interest in diabetes in the young and was Secretary to the Scottish Study Group for the Care of the Young Diabetic from 1990 to 2000.

Bruce Guthrie is Professor of Primary Care at the University of Dundee and is interested in the definition and measurement of quality of health care and the intersection between clinical or technical quality and patient experience of care and caring.

Gill Haddow is a medical sociologist and researcher, based in the ESRC INNOGEN Centre at Edinburgh University. Currently, she is consulting members of the public about some of the ethical, legal and social issues around Generation Scotland, Scotland's first population DNA database.

Alexandra Howson initially trained as a Registered Nurse before becoming a sociologist. She is a researcher, educator and editor with two decades of experience in health and education settings and has held faculty positions at the Universities of Edinburgh, Aberdeen and Abertay, Dundee. She is the author of books and papers on the sociology of the body, gender and health and in 2005 she was a Visiting Scholar at the University of California Berkeley. She currently lives in Washington state and operates as an independent research and editorial consultant at www.thistleeditorial.com.

Guro Huby is CIHR (Centre for Integrated Healthcare Research) Reader in the School of Health in Social Science, University of Edinburgh. CIHR is one of three Scottish Collaborations between NHS organisations and Higher Education Institutions for Nurses, Midwives and Allied Health Professions and works to increase research capacity and capability among nurses, midwives and allied health professionals in Scotland. Before taking up her present post she led the Scotland-wide initiative 'Research-Based Development of Scottish Primary Care.' Health service reform and modernisation, service integration and use of evidence in organizational development and change are key interests, together with development of effective models of knowledge transfer.

Alex Law is a Lecturer in Sociology at the University of Abertay Dundee. His research interests include social movements, the sociology of welfare work, and critical theory. He recently edited a collection with Gerry Mooney, *New Labour/Hard Labour* (Policy Press, 2007), on the changing nature of work in U.K. welfarism and is collaborating on a book on *Social Movements and Social Policy* for Policy Press (forthcoming, 2008).

Guido Möllering is a Researcher at the Max Planck Institute for the Study of Societies in Cologne, Germany. He holds a Ph.D. in Management Studies from the University of Cambridge, United Kingdom. His research is generally in the area of interorganizational relationships and the constitution of markets with specific interests in trust and collective institutional entrepreneurship. He has published numerous articles and book chapters on trust, some of them in leading journals such as *Organization Science* and *Sociology*. He is the author of the book *Trust: Reason, Routine, Reflexivity,* published by Elsevier in 2006.

Peter McKiernan is Professor of Management, and Dean of the School of Management, at the University of St. Andrews. Previously, he was Convenor of the Strategy and Marketing Group, Director of the Full-time MBA and Professor of Strategic Management at Warwick Business School. Peter has published widely in strategic management, including two volumes on the historical development of the discipline and the best-selling book on transformational change—*Sharpbenders* (Basil Blackwell, 1988). His scholarship has won prizes from the BAM, IBM, the British Diabetes Association and Scottish Enterprise.

Hester Parr is a Reader in Social Geography at the University of Dundee and has extensive research interests in community mental health. She has coedited *Mind and Body Spaces* (1999, Routledge) and has numerous articles in *Society and Space, Cultural Geographies, Transactions of the Institute of British Geographers*. Her monograph *Mental Health and Social Space: Towards Inclusionary Geographies?* is to be published in 2008 by Blackwell.

Valerie M. Sheach Leith is a Lecturer in Sociology at The Robert Gordon University, Aberdeen. Her research and teaching interests include the sociology of the body, qualitative research methods and trust relationships in the health care setting.

Marit Solbjør, is a sociologist at the Norwegian University of Science and Technology (NTNU). She did her Ph.D. project on women's experiences of mammography screening at the Department of Public Health and General Practice, NTNU. She is currently working as a researcher at NTNU, studying user involvement in hospital settings.

Irena Stepanikova is an Assistant Professor in the Department of Sociology at the University of South Carolina. Her research interests include social psychology, racial and ethnic relations, and medical sociology. She currently studies the roles of race and ethnicity in physician–patient interaction.

Index

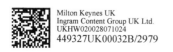

Milton Keynes UK
Ingram Content Group UK Ltd.
UKHW020028071024
449327UK00032B/2979